Department of Health and Social Security
Ministry of Agriculture, Fisheries and Food
Scottish Home and Health Department
Department of Agriculture and Fisheries for Scotland
Welsh Office
Department of Health and Social Services for Nor
Department of Agriculture for Northern Irelan

Guide to

Good Pharmaceutical Manufacturing Practice 1983

Editor: J R Sharp

London
Her Majesty's Stationery Office

First published 1971
Second edition 1977
Third edition 1983
Fourth impression 1987

ISBN 0 11 320832 4

CONTENTS

PREFACE

This Guide was compiled by the Medicines Inspectorate of the Department of Health and Social Security in consultation with other interested bodies. It has no statutory force and should not be regarded as an interpretation of the requirements of any Act, Regulation or Directive. Its purpose is to recommend steps which should be taken, as necessary and appropriate, by manufacturers of medicinal products with the object of ensuring that their products are of the nature and quality intended.

It is recognised that there are acceptable methods, other than those described in this guide, which are capable of achieving the same objectives.

The Guide is particularly concerned with those aspects of quality, safety and efficacy which may be affected by manufacturing processes carried out on any scale, and sets out principles applicable to such processes. It is not, except indirectly, concerned with the safety of persons connected with the manufacture of medicinal products. It should not be read as augmenting, or causing dispute with, anything issued by the Health and Safety Executive.

A Glossary of Terms, as used in this Guide, is included to avoid possible ambiguity. Although a reference is made to the Medicines Act (1968) definition of 'Medicinal Product', the other definitions are not intended to be legal definitions.

INTRODUCTION

The first edition of the 'Guide to Good Pharmaceutical Manufacturing Practice' was published in 1971, before any formal inspections of pharmaceutical manufacturers had been carried out under the Medicines Act. It was therefore written at a time when the nature, extent, and special problems of the manufacture of medicinal products in the United Kingdom were not completely known. Nevertheless, those who drafted that first edition had made a number of informal visits to manufacturers, and they were able to draw both on their own industrial experience, and on a number of other national and international GMP codes, guides and regulations.

The first edition, published only after extensive consultation with interested official, industrial, professional and academic bodies, rapidly came to be acknowledged as 'a collection of principles of known and accepted good practice'. Because of the colour of its cover it became known as 'The Orange Guide'.

In 1977 a second edition was published, following wider experience of medicines manufacture which had suggested that some expansion and clarification would be useful. The whole text was revised, some entirely new sections added, and similar extensive consultation procedures were followed. At the same time, thought was given to frequency of revision and it was decided that, whilst a revision would not necessarily be published every five years, the existing edition should at least be considered for revision at approximately five-year intervals. Consideration of the second edition, five years on, led to the conclusion that a revision could usefully be undertaken, hence this third edition. It is published in the same spirit as the earlier editions, as a work of guidance, produced in consultation, rather than as a set of inflexible rules.

Time has shown that it would be helpful to re-arrange and, in places, clarify and enlarge the text, and to give guidance on further topics. The text is now restructured in three main parts. Part I (Sections 1 to 8) covers matters of general concern and application to the manufacture and control of *all* medicines, and thus establishes general GMP principles and guidelines. Part II (Sections 9–13) gives additional guidance specific to various major categories of production, and Part III (Sections 14–18) deals with a number of more specialised topics. One of the effects of this re-arrangement is that important topics such as the manufacture of Sterile Products cease to be mere appendices. Also, with the removal of the former 'Introduction' (now the 'Preface') outside the section-numbering scheme and the transfer of the expanded Glossary to the rear, the section on 'Quality' becomes, fittingly, 'Part I, Section 1'.

Significant changes or additions include:

a. Some additional paragraphs under 'Documentation' dealing with electromagnetic and Photographic Records. (3.45 to 3.49)
b. Additional material on Storage Areas under 'Premises'. (4.23 to 4.29)
c. Some further explanatory comment on cross contamination. (5.13 and Appendix 2)
d. An expansion of the sub-sections dealing with the receipt, sampling, testing, storage and dispensing of starting materials. (5.14 to 5.25 and Appendix 4)
e. Expansion of the advice given on avoidance of labelling errors. (5.38 and Appendix 5)
f. Guidance on Returned Goods under 'Recovered Materials'. (6.7 to 6.8)
g. Expansion of the section on 'Product Recall' to cover Complaints Procedures. (Section 7)
h. Re-writing of the section on 'Good Laboratory Practice' (now 'Good Control Laboratory Practice'). (Section 8)
i. Partial re-writing, and considerable re-arrangement, of the section on Sterile Product Manufacture. (Section 9)
j. Expansion of the section on 'Contract Manufacture' to cover, in addition, Contract Analysis and Service Contracts. (Section 14)

Entirely new sections are:

11. Liquids, Creams and Ointments
12. Medical Gases
13. Radiopharmaceuticals
14. Veterinary Medicines
15. Electronic Data Processing

Some appendices have been added (of which those on Basic Environmental Standards for the Manufacture of Sterile Products and on Certificates of Analysis in particular contain new material) together with a bibliography and an index.

Although the word 'must' is occasionally used for special emphasis, the favoured form throughout is to describe what 'should' be done. This has at times caused some doubts over interpretation, most especially overseas, where some languages do not include both the 'should' and 'must' forms, or where different significances are attached to these words. The principle adopted for this Guide is that the more emphatic 'must' form is generally inappropriate in what is, in fact a *guide*. Where 'should' is used, it is to be taken in the sense that 'it is Good Manufacturing Practice to . . .' or, alternatively, '. . . this is an acceptable way of complying with the principles of GMP'.

Another difficulty in interpretation which is occasionally encountered is over the use of 'absolute' terms (such as 'ensure that . . .', 'eliminate', 'avoid', 'absence of . . .') and the difficulty of requiring, proving or demonstrating, an absolute. Since the avoidance of such terms can lead to lack of emphasis or tiresome circumlocution, they are used in this Guide with the intention of being interpreted only in a rationally practical manner. Thus, such phrases as 'to ensure that . . .' or 'to eliminate . . .' are to be read as meaning 'to ensure that (or to eliminate etc) *as far as is reasonably practicable*'.

Whilst there is a certain amount of repetition (both for the sake of emphasis, and also to aid in directing the reader to matters relevant to a given topic under other headings), it must also be appreciated that a publication such as this could not possibly cover every facet of good practice in the manufacture of medicinal products. The absence of any specific statement in this Guide should not be taken to condone the commission or omission of any practice, should rational considerations dictate otherwise.

Earlier consultation drafts suggested the inclusion of an Appendix giving tentative microbial monitoring standards for Sterile Products Areas. Widely canvassed opinion was almost equally divided for and against the inclusion of such an appendix, but amongst those in favour there was no uniformity of opinion as to what the *published* standards should be. In the circumstances, only figures as given for viable organism count in the Pharmaceutical Inspection Convention Annex on the Manufacture of Sterile Products (PH 1/81 of May 1981) have been included. (See Appendix 1 of this Guide). This however, does not imply any under-valuing of the importance of microbiological monitoring in Aseptic, Clean and other areas.

The object of GMP and any guide to it is, initially, the assurance of the quality of the product, and ultimately the safety, well-being and protection of the patient. The essence of this Guide is contained in the first section, 'Quality'. In a sense, the rest is merely an expansion of, or series of footnotes, to it.

The term 'quality' has a variety of 'dictionary' definitions in addition to the more specialised senses in which it is used in Statistical Quality Control. In this Guide the word is used in the sense both of the essential nature of a thing, and also of the totality of its attributes and properties which bear upon its fitness for its intended purpose. The basic concept is that Assurance of that required Quality cannot be achieved by the testing of end-product samples alone. Whilst certain more general inferences may be drawn from the results of such testing, a full understanding and evaluation of the *total* quality of the *total* batch may only be embraced by a consideration of many other factors, that is by and through a system of *Quality Assurance*. This and other related terms are defined in the first section, where it will be seen that 'Quality Assurance' embraces 'Good Manufacturing Practice' as well as other factors such as original product design and development. 'Quality Control' in turn is but part of 'Good Manufacturing Practice' but nevertheless is considerably broader in scope than the laboratory testing of samples.

It is impossible to over-emphasise the importance of *people*, at all levels, in the Assurance of the Quality of medicinal products. The great majority of defective medicinal products reported result simply from human error or carelessness, not from failures in technology. The designation of any person, section or department as 'Quality Assurance' or 'Quality Control' should increase, rather than reduce or supplant, the sense of responsibility for quality in other persons and departments within the organisation.

ACKNOWLEDGEMENTS

The original drafts of this Guide were prepared by the Medicines Inspectorate: K.J. Ayling B Pharm, MPS, R. Baker PhD, B Pharm, BSc (Econ) FPS, FBIM, D.I.R. Begg MPS, FIQA, B.A. Curran BSc (Pharm), P.D. Evans BSc (Pharm) MPS, J. Flint FPS, MInst Pkg, H.F. Gough MSc, CChem, FRSC, MBIM, D. Haythornthwaite B Pharm MPS, W.J. Hewlett BSc, CChem, MRSC, R.C. Hutton PhD, BSc, CChem, FRSC, D.E. Jenkins B Pharm, MPS, DMS, MBIM, A.J. Middleton B Pharm, MPS, CChem, FRSC, MPhA, D.P. Mogg MSc, AMBIM, P.A. Ramskir BSc, CChem, FRSC, AMBIM, J.R. Sharp BSc, CChem, FRSC, FIQA, J.A. Thomson BSc, CChem, MRSC, J.L. Turner B Pharm, MPS, DMS, D.R.S. Warburton CChem, MRSC, ACT, I.E. Williams B Pharm, MPS, GIChem E, M.G. Willows MPS, FRSH.

Also from within DHSS most valuable comments and suggestions were received from: J.P. Griffin PhD, MB, BS, BSc, MRCS, MRCP, J.A. Holgate MB, ChB, MSc, FIBiol, C.A. Johnson B Pharm, BSc, FPS, CChem, FRSC, MPhA, A.G. Stewart M Phil, MPS, W.G. Thomas MSc, PhD, FPS, B.A. Wills B Pharm, PhD, FPS, CChem, FRSC.

A consultation draft was circulated for comment to interested organisations, bodies and persons. Whilst it is not possible to acknowledge all the many responses, particular thanks are due to the following organisations, with which extensive and most constructive discussions were held:
The Association of the British Pharmaceutical Industry, as represented by its Good Manufacturing Practices Sub-Committee:
J.F. Chissell MSc (Chairman), M. Bennoson B Tech, CChem, MRSC, G. Drewery BSc, M Chem A, CChem, FRSC, R.E.M. Heskell MPS, S.M. Murray B Tech, CChem, FRSC, N.J. Phipps, CChem, MRSC, T.I. Richardson BSc.

Especial thanks are due to Messrs Chissell and Drewery and to M. Murray BSc (Pharm) MPS (Technical Services Manager, ABPI) who acted as spokesmen for the above sub-committee.

The Pharmaceutical Quality Group of the Institute of Quality Assurance, as represented by:
P. Atherton ARTCS, CChem, FRSC, FIQA, E.R. Evans MIQA, M.Inst.Pkg, A.C. Harper CChem, MRSC, FIQA, I.A. Martin BSc, PhD, S.J. Pratt ARCS, PhD, MRSC, FIQA, C.D. Ratcliffe BSc, CChem, FRSC, FIQA, A.A. Wagland BSc, PhD, FIQA.

The Proprietary Association of Great Britain, as represented by its GMP Working Party:
J.P. Beaumont BSc, CChem, MRSC, A. Gaskell PhC, FPS, I.A. Martin BSc, PhD, D.M. Merrington B Pharm, MPS, Marion Kelly MPS, A.D. Smith CChem, MRSC, W.G. Whittington B Pharm, FPS.

Other bodies which provided valuable and constructive comment included:
Blood Products Laboratory, Estree
British Oxygen Company
The Company Chemists Association
The European Organisation for Quality Control
Leeds Area Health Authority
The Medicines Testing Laboratory, Edinburgh
Ministry of Agriculture Fisheries and Food
The Pharmaceutical Society of Great Britain
The Regional Pharmaceutical Officers Committee
The Royal Society of Chemistry
The Scottish Home and Health Department
The Scottish Pharmaceutical Sciences Group
South West Thames Regional Health Authority
The Welsh Office

Thanks are also due to the following individuals for their comments and advice:
A.J. Badby BSc, CChem, FRSC, MBIM, W.A. Bennett MA, PhD, E.G. Beveridge B Pharm, PhD, PhC, MPS, T.J. Bradley BSc, PhD, FPS, MIBiol, R. Feakes LRSC, R. Dickinson FPS, MCPP. S.P. Denyer B Pharm, PhD, MPS, G. Farquharson BSc, MCIBS, J.W. Hemingway BSc, MInst P, J.A.J. Goldsmith BSc, PhD, CChem, FRSC, FIQA, C.R. Hitchings B Pharm, MSc, MPS, MCPP, B.A. Henman DMS, FBIM, CChem, MRSC, H.T. Hoskins MSc, MPS, MIPhM, I. Martin BSc, DCC, MIBiol, FIQA, B. Mullock PhD, CChem, FRSC, FBIM, D. Pullen, M.I.Mech E, I.K. Sykes PhD, BSc, A.J. Trill MSc, B Pharm, MPS, MBIM, J.P. Wells FPS, G. Zajicek B Pharm, MPS.

The Editor would also like to express his personal thanks to Dave Begg for suggesting a design for the cover, to Mike Willows for his assistance in sorting and collating written comments, to Sheila Shrigley for her advice on the Bibliography, and to Mrs Ronan and her word-processing ladies (Carol and Virginia) of the DHSS Typing Pool, Market Towers, for so nobly coping with a complex series of barely legible manuscript amendments to amended amendments.

J.R.S.

Part One

1. QUALITY

PRINCIPLE

There should be a comprehensive system, so designed, documented, implemented and controlled, and so furnished with personnel, equipment and other resources as to provide assurance that products will be consistently of a quality appropriate to their intended use. The attainment of this quality objective requires the involvement and commitment of all concerned, at all stages.

Note on Terminology

To avoid confusion, and in order to clarify their inter-relationships, the terms 'Quality Assurance', 'Quality Control', and 'Good Manufacturing Practice' are defined here rather than in the Glossary. The basic concepts adopted for this Guide are:

Quality Assurance

Is the sum total of the organised arrangements made with the object of ensuring that products will be of the quality required by their intended use. It is Good Manufacturing Practice *plus* factors outside the scope of this Guide (such as original product design and development).

Good Manufacturing Practice

Is that part of Quality Assurance aimed at ensuring that products are consistently manufactured to a quality appropriate to their intended use. It is thus concerned with both Manufacturing and Quality Control procedures.

Quality Control

Is that part of Good Manufacturing Practice which is concerned with sampling, specification and testing, and with the organisation, documentation and release procedures which ensure that the necessary and relevant tests are, in fact, carried out, and that materials are not released for use, nor products released for sale or supply, until their quality has been judged to be satisfactory. ['Quality Control' is sometimes used in the sense of the organisational entity which has responsibility for these functions.]

(The word 'system' is used in the 'Principle' above in the sense of a regulated pattern of interacting activities and techniques which are united to form an organised whole.)

QUALITY ASSURANCE

1.1 The objectives of Quality Assurance are achieved when processes have been defined which, when followed, will yield a product that complies with its specification, and when the finished product:

(a) contains the correct ingredients in the correct proportions

(b) has been correctly processed, according to the defined procedures

(c) is of the purity required

(d) is enclosed in its proper container, which

(e) bears the correct label (or is otherwise suitably marked or identified) and

(f) is stored, distributed and subsequently handled so that its quality is maintained throughout its designated or expected life.

GOOD MANUFACTURING PRACTICE

1.2 The basic requirements of Good Manufacturing Practice are that:

(a) All manufacturing processes should be clearly defined, and known to be capable of achieving the desired ends.

(b) all necessary facilities are provided, including:

- (i) appropriately trained personnel
- (ii) adequate premises and space
- (iii) suitable equipment and services
- (iv) correct materials, containers and labels
- (v) approved procedures (including cleaning procedures)
- (vi) suitable storage and transport.

(c) procedures are written in instructional form, in clear and unambiguous language, and are specifically applicable to the facilities provided.

(d) operators are trained to carry out the procedures correctly.

(e) records are made during manufacture (including packaging) which demonstrate that all the steps required by the defined procedures were, *in fact* taken and that the quantity and quality produced were those expected.

(f) records of manufacture and distribution which enable the complete history of a batch to be traced, are retained in a legible and accessible form.

(g) a system is available to recall from sale or supply any batch or product, should that become necessary.

QUALITY CONTROL

1.3 To achieve effective control of Quality:

(a) Adequate facilities and staff should be available for sampling, inspecting and testing starting materials, packaging materials, intermediate, bulk and finished products, and where appropriate, for determining environmental quality.

(b) Samples of starting materials, packaging materials, intermediate products, bulk products and finished products should only be taken by personnel and methods approved by the person responsible for Quality Control.

(c) Results of the inspection and testing of materials, and of intermediate, bulk or finished products should be formally assessed against specification by the person responsible for Quality Control (or a person designated by him) before products are released for sale or supply.

Product assessment should include a review and evaluation of relevant manufacturing (including packaging) documentation.

(d) Sufficient reference samples of starting materials and products should be retained (the latter, where possible, in the final pack) to permit future examination if necessary.

Self Inspection

1.4 Measures should be taken to confirm that designated Manufacturing and Quality Assurance procedures are being followed by staff at all levels. To this end appropriate Production, Quality Control and (as necessary) Engineering staff should carry-out periodic inspection and evaluation of the Company's own Quality Assurance systems. This should cover production, warehousing and quality control laboratories, and result in a formal written report with recommendations for action. Follow-up action should be recorded.

2. PERSONNEL AND TRAINING

PRINCIPLES

There should be sufficient personnel at all levels with the ability, training, experience and, where necessary, the professional/technical qualifications and managerial skills appropriate to the tasks assigned to them. Their duties and responsibilities should be clearly explained to them and recorded as written job descriptions or by other suitable means. Training should cover not only specific tasks but Good Manufacturing Practice generally and the importance of personal hygiene.

General

2.1 The key personnel are the person responsible for Production and the person responsible for Quality Control, who should be different persons, neither of whom should be responsible to the other, but who both have a responsibility for achieving the requisite quality.

[Note – The duties of the person responsible for Quality Control are wider than those which may be suggested by such terms as 'Chief Analyst', 'Laboratory Head' etc].

2.2 Persons in responsible positions should have sufficient authority to discharge their responsibilities. In particular, the person responsible for Quality Control should be able to carry out his defined functions impartially.

2.3 Only in exceptional circumstances should persons engaged part-time or in a consultative capacity be appointed to key positions.

2.4 Persons should be designated to take up the duties of key personnel during the absence of the latter.

2.5 Key personnel should be provided with adequate supporting staff.

Distribution of Key Responsibilities

2.6 The way in which the various key responsibilities which can influence product quality are distributed may vary with different manufacturers. These responsibilities should be clearly defined and allocated.

2.7 The person responsible for Quality Control should have the authority to establish, verify and implement all quality control procedures. He should have the authority, independent of Production, to approve materials and products, and to reject as he sees fit starting materials, packaging materials and intermediate, bulk and finished products which do not comply with the relevant specification, or which were not manufactured in accordance with the approved methods and under the prescribed conditions. (His authority in relation to packaging materials may be limited to those which may influence product quality, identity, and safety in use).

2.8 The Production Manager, in addition to his responsibilities for production areas, equipment, operations and records; for the management of production personnel; and for the manufacture of products in accordance with the appropriate Master Formula and Method, will have other responsibilities bearing on quality which he should share, or exercise jointly, with the person responsible for Quality Control.

2.9 These shared or joint responsibilities may include authorising written procedures; monitoring and control of the manufacturing environment; plant cleanliness; process validation; training of personnel; approval of suppliers of materials and of contract acceptors; protection of products and material against spoilage and deterioration; retention of records. It is important that both direct and shared responsibilities are understood by those concerned.

Training

2.10 All Production, Quality Control and Laboratory personnel and all other personnel (e.g. maintenance, service and cleaning staff) whose duties take them into manufacturing areas, or which bear upon manufacturing activities, should be trained in the principles of Good Manufacturing Practice and in the practice (and the relevant theory) of the tasks assigned to them.

2.11 Training should be in accordance with written programmes approved by the person responsible for Production and, as appropriate, by the person responsible for Quality Control. Special attention should be given to training of operators working in aseptic or clean areas, or with highly potent, toxic, or sensitising materials.

2.12 Training should be given at recruitment, and be augmented and revised as necessary. Training records should be maintained and periodic assessments of the effectiveness of training programmes should be made.

Checks should be carried out to confirm that designated procedures are being followed by staff at all levels.

Hygiene

2.13 High standards of personal cleanliness should be observed by all those concerned with production processes. (The special requirements for Sterile Products are covered in Section 9).

2.14 Hand-washing and hygienic drying facilities should be conveniently available to, and used by, manufacturing personnel. (Such facilities should not be sited within aseptic areas, see Section 9.34).

2.15 All persons entering production areas should wear protective garments, including headgear, appropriate to the processes being carried out. The garments should be regularly and frequently cleaned and not worn outside the factory premises. Changing Rooms should be provided.

2.16 Direct contact should be avoided between the operators' hands and starting materials, intermediates and products (other than when they are in closed containers).

2.17 There should be pre-employment medical checks, and steps should be taken to see that no person with a disease in a communicable form, or with open lesions on the exposed surface of the body, is engaged in the manufacture of medicinal products.

2.18 Staff should be required to report infections and skin lesions, and a defined procedure followed when they are reported. Supervisory staff should look for the signs and symptoms of these conditions.

2.19 Eating, drinking, chewing and smoking, or the storage of food, drink, smoking material and personal medication should not be permitted within manufacturing areas or in any other area where they might adversely influence product quality.

[NOTE – Requirements regarding personal hygiene and protective clothing apply to all persons (including visitors, maintenance personnel, senior management and Inspectors) entering production areas.]

3. DOCUMENTATION

PRINCIPLES

Documentation is a prime necessity in Quality Assurance. Its purposes are to define the system of control, to reduce the risk of error inherent in purely oral communication, to ensure that personnel are instructed in the details of, and follow, the procedures concerned, and to permit investigation and tracing of defective products. The system of documentation should be such that the history of each batch of product, including the utilisation and disposal of starting materials, packaging materials and intermediate, bulk and finished products, may be determined.

General

3.1 To facilitate proper and effective use of documents they should be designed and prepared with care, and with particular attention to the following points:

(a) The title (which should be unambiguous), nature and purpose of the document should be clearly stated. The document should be laid out in an orderly fashion, and be easy to check. Where a document has been revised systems should be operated to prevent inadvertent use of superseded documents.

(b) It is an advantage if it is possible to revise part of a document without necessarily completely rewriting the whole.

(c) The way the document is to be used, and by whom, should be clearly apparent from the document itself. Other means provided to explain its use are of less value.

(d) Where documents bear instructions they should be written in the imperative, as numbered steps. They should be clear, precise, unambiguous and in language the user can understand. Such documents should be readily available to all concerned with carrying out the instructions.

(e) Documents which require the entry of data should:

- (i) Provide sufficient space for the entry
- (ii) Allow adequate spacing between entries
- (iii) Show headings clearly indicating what is to be entered.

(f) Persons making entries should do so in clear legible writing, and should confirm the entry by adding their initials or signatures. A signed recorded observation is preferable to simply ticking in a box.

(g) Manuscript entries should be made in ink or other indelible medium.

(h) The size and shape of documents and the quality and colour of the paper used should be considered in relation to the typing/printing, reproduction and filing facilities available.

(i) Reproduced documents should be clear and legible.

3.2 Documents should contain all necessary, but no superfluous data. Any headings, or places for entries, which cease to be used should be removed at the earliest opportunity.

3.3 If an error is made or detected on a document it should be corrected in such a manner that the original entry is not lost and the correction initialled and dated. Where appropriate, the reason for the correction should be recorded.

3.4 Documents should be kept up to date. Any amendments should be formally authorised and signed. In the case of permanent amendments, the amended document should be replaced at the earliest opportunity by a newly prepared document.

3.5 The documentation system should include provision for periodic review and revision as necessary.

3.6 An out-dated or superseded document should be removed from active use, and a copy retained for reference.

3.7 It may be useful to prepare a manual which describes the overall Quality Assurance system, the procedures employed and the documents used.

Specifications: Starting Materials

3.8 There should be a Specification, approved by the person responsible for Quality Control, for each starting material.

3.9 Each Specification should be dated and include:

(a) A designated name, with reference to monograph specifications where appropriate, and, preferably, a code reference unique to the material.

(b) A reference to any alternative proprietary designation of the material.

(c) A description of the physical form of the material.

(d) Sampling instructions.

(e) Tests and limits for identity, purity, physical and chemical characteristics, microbiological standards (where appropriate) and assay.

(f) Details of, or reference to, the test methods to be used to assess identity and quality, and to perform the assay.

(g) Approved supplier(s) of the material.

(h) Safety precautions to be observed.

(i) Storage conditions.

(j) Frequency of re-testing the stored material.

[NOTE – Certain of these requirements may not necessarily appear on the prime specification document. There may be, for example, standard company sampling procedures and lists of approved suppliers to which the specification explicitly, or by implication, refers.]

Specifications: Packaging Materials

3.10 There should be Packaging Material Specifications, approved by the person responsible for Quality Control.

3.11 Each Specification should be dated and include:

(a) A designated name, with preferably a code-reference unique to the material. This reference should also appear on printed materials.

(b) A description of the nature, dimensions and material of construction of the component with quality standards, control limits, mould references, drawings and details of text, as applicable.

(c) Details of tests for determining compliance with the Specification.

(d) Details of approved suppliers of the component.

(e) Instructions for sampling.

(f) Storage conditions.

(g) Frequency of re-inspection of the stored component.

[NOTE – (i) Certain of these requirements may not necessarily appear on the prime specification document. See Note under 'Starting Material Specification' above.

(ii) See definition of 'Packaging Material' in Glossary. The need for detailed specifications may not apply to 'Other Packaging Materials'.]

3.12 A file of reference specimens of current printed packaging materials should be maintained.

Specifications: Intermediates and Bulk Products

3.13 These Specifications should, as appropriate, be similar to Finished Product Specifications.

Specifications: Finished Products

3.14 There should be specifications, approved by the person responsible for Quality Control, defining the nature and quality of each finished product.

3.15 Each Specification should be dated and include:

(a) The designated name of the product.

(b) A description of the physical form of the product and a reference to container and package details.

(c) Sampling instructions.

(d) Tests and limits for identity, purity, physical and chemical characteristics, microbiological standards (where appropriate) and assay, with details of (or reference to) the test-methods to be used.

(e) Safety precautions to be observed.

(f) Storage conditions.

(g) Frequency of re-examination of the stored product.

[NOTE – Certain of these requirements may not necessarily appear on the prime document. See Note under 'Starting Material Specifications' above.]

Sampling and Approval Documentation

3.16 There should be documentary systems set up with the object of ensuring that:

(a) Starting and Packaging Materials are in fact sampled and tested in accordance with previously specified procedures.

(b) Materials are not taken into usable stock until the specified checks and tests have been performed and the material formally approved by Quality Control. (Alternative arrangements may be made when an acceptable certificate of analysis is available – see Appendix 3).

(c) Intermediate, bulk and finished products, and any re-worked or recovered materials, *are* sampled and tested in accordance with previously defined procedures, and that products will not be released for sale or supply until all data on the intermediate, bulk and finished product have been reviewed, and approval given, by Quality Control.

Master Formula and Method

3.17 A formally authorised Master Formula and Method should exist for each product and batch size to be manufactured.

3.18 *The Master Formula* should be dated and include:

(a) The name of the product, with a code reference relating it to its Specification.

(b) A description of the pharmaceutical form and strength of the product.

(c) A list of all starting materials to be used (see 3.19) with the amount of each, whether or not they appear in the Finished Product. All quantities should be stated in a uniform system of measurement, with a statement of any calculated overage. Where material of variable potency is to be used the permissible limits of variation and the total potency required for a batch should be stated.

(d) A statement of the total expected final yield, and of relevant intermediate yields.

3.19 Each starting material should be designated in the Master Formula by:

(a) The Approved or Monograph Name, and/or any other descriptive name, by which it can be specifically identified, and which is used whenever that material is referred to.

(b) A code reference which is unique to that material.

3.20 *The Method* should be dated and, as appropriate, include:

(a) A statement of the manufacturing location and the equipment to be used.

(b) The methods, or reference to the methods, to be used for preparing the equipment (eg cleaning, assembling, calibrating, sterilising).

(c) Detailed stepwise processing instructions, including:

- (i) A check that the materials used are those intended.
- (ii) Any required pre-treatment of materials.
- (iii) Sequences for adding materials.
- (iv) Mixing times (as appropriate).
- (v) Temperatures (as relevant).
- (vi) Safety precautions to be observed.

(d) A statement of the theoretical and/or expected amount of product at pertinent stages of manufacture.

(e) Details of any in-process controls, with instructions for sampling and with control limits.

(f) Requirements for bulk storage of the product, including containers, labels and special storage conditions.

(See also Section 6 regarding documentation of product residue and re-work usage).

Master Packaging Instruction

3.21 A formally authorised Master Packaging Instruction should exist for each pack size and type. It should be dated and (as appropriate) include, or have a reference to:

(a) The name of the product.

(b) A description of its pharmaceutical form and strength.

(c) The pack size expressed as number, weight or volume of the product in the final container.

(d) A complete list with quantities, sizes and types of all the packaging materials required.

(e) The code or reference number of each material which relates it to its Specification.

(f) A specimen or facsimile of relevant printed packaging material, where practicable.

(g) A description of the packaging operation with an indication of the equipment to be used.

(h) Details of any required preparation of packaging materials (eg washing, blowing, sterilising) and of any over-printing necessary.

(i) Special precautions to be observed.

(j) Details of any in-process controls to be applied, with instructions for sampling and with control limits.

[NOTES – (i) It is useful to be able to refer to superseded Master Packaging Instructions.

(ii) Where products may be stored in a partially packaged form, requirements for such storage should be laid-down in the Master Documentation, or for example, in standard procedures.]

Records: Starting Materials

3.22 The receipt of each delivery of each starting material should be recorded. The record should include:

(a) Date of receipt.

(b) Name of Material.

(c) Name of material on delivery note and/or containers – if different from (b).

(d) Supplier's name.

(e) Supplier's batch or reference number.

(f) Total quantity, and number of containers received.

(g) The batch identifying number assigned on, or after, receipt.

3.23 The testing of each starting material should be recorded. The record should include:

(a) Date of testing.

(b) Name of material.

(c) The batch identifying number.

(d) Results of all tests.

(e) Identity of person(s) who performed tests.

(f) A cross reference to any relevant Certificate of analysis. (See Appendix 3.)

(g) The signed release or rejection (or other status decision) by Quality Control.

(h) A clear statement of the assigned potency where this can vary.

[NOTE – It is useful to record analytical data in a manner that will facilitate comparative reviews of past results and the detection of trends.]

3.24 Stock records should be maintained of starting materials that will permit stock reconciliations to be made.

3.25 A sample of the starting material sufficient in size to permit analytical re-examination should be retained as part of the starting material record.

Records: Packaging Materials

3.26 The receipt of each delivery of each packaging material should be recorded. The record should include:

(a) Date of receipt.

(b) Name of material.

(c) Supplier's name and any reference or batch number.

(d) Quantity received.

(e) Any batch identifying number assigned on, or after, receipt.

3.27 The testing and inspection of packaging materials should be recorded. The record should include:

(a) Date of testing (or inspection).

(b) Name of material.

(c) The batch identifying number.

(d) Results of testing and inspection.

(e) Name of person(s) who carried out testing or inspection.

(f) The signed release or rejection (or other status decision) by Quality Control.

[NOTE – It is useful to record these data in a manner that will facilitate comparative reviews of past results and the detection of trends.]

3.28 Stock records should be maintained of packaging materials that will permit stock reconciliations to be made. (See also note following 5.31 and 'Packaging Materials' in Glossary).

Records: Contract Manufacture

3.29 In-coming materials, part-processed or finished products from contract acceptors should be treated and documented as for Starting Materials.

Batch Manufacturing Records

3.30 Batch Manufacturing Records should carry a batch reference number, and be based upon the currently approved version of the Master Formula and Method. The method of preparation should be designed to avoid transcription errors. Photocopying or some similar method of preparing the basic document is to be preferred.

3.31 If Batch Manufacturing Records do not include complete details of the Method, the operator must have ready access to the currently approved Method.

3.32 Before any manufacture proceeds there should be recorded checks that the equipment and work-station are clear of previous products and documents, and of materials not required for the process in hand, and that equipment is clean and suitable for use.

3.33 During manufacture the following should be entered onto the Batch Manufacturing Record, at the time that each action is taken:

(a) The batch identifying number of each of the starting materials used.

(b) Where the Master Formula permits variation in the quantity of starting material, a record of the amount actually used.

(c) Dates of commencement and completion of manufacture and of significant intermediate stages.

(d) Where more than one batch of a given starting material is used, a record of the actual amount of each batch.

(e) The batch identifying number and amount of any recovered or re-work material added.

(f) The initials of the person(s) who weighed or measured each material and the initials of the person(s) who checked each of these operations, this check being not only of the quantity but also of the labelled identity and batch number of the material.

(The need for the second series of check initials may diminish if equally effective electronic, and other supporting systems are in operation.)

(g) The amount of product obtained at pertinent intermediate stages of manufacture.

(h) The initials of the person responsible for each critical stage of manufacture.

(i) The results of all in-process controls, with the initials of the person(s) carrying them out.

(j) Reference to the precise items of major equipment used, where several of the same type are available for use (i.e. where equipment is replicated). This information may be recorded in 'Plant Usage Logs'.

(k) Details of, and signed authorisation for, any deviation from the Master Formula and Method.

(l) The final batch yield and the number of bulk containers.

(m) Signed agreement by the process supervisor that apart from any deviation noted as in (k) above, manufacture has proceeded in accordance with the Master Formula and Method, and that process or yield variations are adequately explained.

Batch Packaging Records

3.34 Batch Packaging Records should be based upon the currently approved version of the Master Packaging Instruction and prepared from it by a method designed to avoid transcription errors (photocopying or some similar method is to be preferred). The Record should bear a batch reference number, which is specific to a particular packaging run. The batch number which appears on the finished product should be this number, or one which may be easily related to it.

[NOTE — The bulk product and packaging reference numbering systems must make it possible to relate a packaging operation to a bulk batch *and* the bulk batch to any packaging operation(s).]

3.35 If the Batch Packaging Records do not include details of the method of packaging, these should be readily available to the operator(s).

3.36 Before any packaging is undertaken checks should be made that each packaging line or station is clear of previous product, packaging components, or records. These checks should be recorded.

3.37 During packaging the following should be entered onto the Batch Packaging Record, at the time that each action is taken:

(a) The batch number of the Bulk Product to be packaged.

(b) Dates of commencement and completion of packaging and of significant intermediate stages.

(c) The initials of the person(s) who issued the bulk product and printed packaging materials, and of the person(s) who confirmed their correct nature and quantities.

(d) The total quantities of the packaging materials used, with a batch identifying reference to primary and printed packaging materials. (See Glossary).

[Specimens of printed packaging materials used should be attached, or alternatively there should be an arrangement which will permit later reference to specimens of the printed packaging materials used].

(e) The results of any in-process controls, together with the initials of the person responsible for carrying them out.

(f) The initials of the persons who carried-out each significant stage of the packaging operation.

(g) A record of the packaging machines, line or area used.

3.38 Records should be kept of the amount of bulk product supplied, printed materials issued, and finished packs produced, in order to permit stock reconciliations.

Intermediate, Bulk and Finished Product Test Records

3.39 These records should include:

(a) The date of manufacture;

(b) The date of testing;

(c) The batch number;

(d) The name of the material;

(e) The tests done, and the results;

(f) The signed release or rejection (or other status-decision) by Quality Control.

[NOTE — The method of recording should facilitate comparative reviews of past results and the detection of trends.]

3.40 A sample of the final packaged product sufficient in size to permit full re-examination as necessary should be retained as part of the record. If this is not practicable or economic (due, for example to an unusually large pack size) then a smaller sample *in a similar type of pack* may be retained (see also 3.43).

Distribution Records

3.41 To facilitate effective recall, records of distribution should be kept showing the name and addresses of all persons to whom the manufacturer supplies a product. (see Section 7).

Complaints Records

3.42 A record should be maintained of all complaints relating to product or packaging quality. This record should show the nature of the complaint, results of investigations and action taken. The record should be maintained in such a manner that significant recurrent complaints can be recognised and appropriate action taken. (see Section 7).

Retention of Records

3.43 Batch Manufacturing and Packaging Records, plus the relevant test records, must be retained for at least 5 years. Finished product samples should be retained at least until the expiry date of the product, or until such time as the batch may no longer be expected to be in stock or in use. Starting material records should be retained for at least 5 years and the samples for a minimum of 2 years (see 3.46–3.50 regarding copy-records). Finished product reference samples should be stored under ambient conditions, or as directed on the label.

Other Documents

3.44 As and where the scale and nature of an operation demands, there should be written procedures covering aspects, not dealt with in the above paragraphs, which could influence the quality of a product. For example:

(a) Cleaning and maintenance of buildings and equipment.

(b) Setting-up and operating manufacturing and packaging equipment.

(c) Maintenance and checking of equipment.

(d) Control of the manufacturing environment, and monitoring it for potential chemical, physical, and biological contamination hazards.

(e) Training of personnel, particularly with regard to the understanding of relevant procedures and hygiene.

(f) The return of unused material to store, and the handling of reject material, and of material suitable for reworking.

In addition, where relevant to the scale of an operation, the maintenance of departmental and equipment logs (ie running, dated records of equipment usage, products manufactured and cleaning of equipment and manufacturing areas) is recommended.

Electromagnetic and Photographic Records

3.45 For guidance on electromagnetic records and storage of data, see Section 16 on Electronic Data Processing.

3.46 The manner of recording data for subsequent copying (by microfilm, microfiche etc) should be such as to ensure that the copying system will reproduce the data clearly and accurately. Type and colour of ink to be used, method of making alterations, and whether or not entries are permitted on reverse sides of documents should all be considered. Adherence to the defined method should be monitored.

3.47 Where interpretation of an original document depends on colour distinction (eg on multiple trace chart records) it must be possible to interpret accurately any black-and-white copy made from it.

3.48 Original documents should be retained for at least six months after the batch to which they relate is first sold or supplied. They should not be destroyed until any copies made from them have been checked against them for completeness and legibility.

3.49 There should be provision for making legible copies of records stored on photographic film.

4. PREMISES AND EQUIPMENT

PRINCIPLES

Buildings should be located, designed, constructed, adapted and maintained to suit the operations carried out in them. Equipment should be designed, constructed, adapted, located and maintained to suit the processes and products for which it is used. Building construction, and equipment lay-out, should ensure protection of the product from contamination, permit efficient cleaning and avoid the accumulation of dust and dirt.

(For additional guidance on premises for Sterile Products Manufacture, see section 9).

4.1 Premises should be sited to avoid contamination from the external environment or from other near-by activities. In existing premises, effective measures should be taken to avoid such contamination.

4.2 Animal houses should be well isolated from manufacturing areas.

4.3 Premises should be constructed and maintained with the object of protecting against weather, ground seepage and the entrance and harbouring of vermin, birds, pests and pets.

4.4 Premises should be designed and laid-out in such a way that the risk of mix-up or contamination of one product or material by another is minimised. This especially applies to premises for the handling of highly toxic or sensitising materials such as hormones, cytotoxic agents and certain antibiotics.

4.5 Protection from the weather should be provided for receiving and despatch areas, and for materials and products in transit.

4.6 Premises should be maintained in a good state of repair. The condition of buildings should be reviewed regularly, and repairs effected where necessary. Special care should be exercised to ensure that building, repair or maintenance operations do not hazard products.

4.7 Premises should provide sufficient space to suit the operations to be carried out, allow an efficient flow of work, and permit effective communication and supervision.

4.8 The processing of materials for non-medicinal use should be appropriately segregated from the processing of medicinal products.

4.9 Cloakrooms should be separate from, or partitioned from, processing areas. Toilets should be well ventilated and not open directly to manufacturing areas.

4.10 Premises in which medicinal products are manufactured or stored should be made secure, with access restricted to authorised personnel. Additional security arrangements may be necessary in specific areas or for specific products.

4.11 Floors in processing areas should be made of impervious materials, laid to an even surface. They should be free from cracks and open joints and should allow prompt and efficient removal of any spillages. Walls should be sound and finished with a smooth, impervious and washable surface. Ceilings should be so constructed and finished that they can be maintained in a clean condition. The coving of junctions between walls, floors and ceilings in critical areas is recommended.

4.12 Pipework, light fittings, ventilation points and other services in manufacturing areas should be sited to avoid creating uncleanable recesses. Services should preferably run outside the processing areas. They should be sealed into any walls and partitions through which they pass.

4.13 Drains should be of adequate size, and should have trapped gullies and proper ventilation. Open channels should be avoided where possible, but if they are necessary they should be shallow to facilitate cleaning and disinfection.

4.14 Buildings should be effectively lit and ventilated, with air control facilities (including temperature, humidity and filtration), appropriate both to the operations undertaken within them and to the external environment.

4.15 Working conditions (e.g. temperature, humidity, noise levels) should be such that there is no adverse effect on the product, either directly or indirectly.

4.16 Air intakes and exhausts, and associated pipework and trunking, should be sited to avoid product contamination hazards.

4.17 Manufacturing areas should not be used as a general right of way for personnel or materials, or for storage (except of materials in process).

4.18 All premises, including processing areas, laboratories, stores, passage ways and external surrounds should be maintained in a clean and tidy condition.

4.19 Waste material should not be allowed to accumulate. It should be collected in suitable receptacles for removal to collection points outside the buildings, and disposed of at regular and frequent intervals. Special care is necessary over the disposal of waste containing dangerous, highly toxic or sensitising materials (eg hormones, cytotoxic agents, sensitising antibiotics). Disposal of raw materials, printed Packaging Materials and rejected products should be carefully controlled and documented.

4.20 There should be written cleaning procedures and schedules for manufacturing and storage areas.

4.21 Vacuum or wet cleaning methods are to be preferred. Compressed air and brushes should be used with care, and avoided if possible, as they increase the risk of product contamination. (For additional guidance on premises for Sterile Products Manufacture, see Section 9.)

4.22 Adequate space (preferably separated from processing areas) should be provided for cleaning and storing mobile equipment, and the storage of cleaning materials.

Storage areas

4.23 Storage areas should be designed, laid-out and be of sufficient capacity to permit effective and orderly segregation of the various categories of material stored, and to allow rotation of stock.

4.24 Segregated storage should be provided for rejected, recalled or returned goods. Where the maintenance of quarantine status depends upon storage in separate areas, such areas should be provided, with restricted access.

4.25 In particular, labels and other printed packaging materials (including labels for starting materials and for bulk and intermediate products) should be stored in a secure manner that will permit issue only to authorised persons in accordance with formal documented procedures. Storage arrangements should permit separation of different labels (and other printed materials) and avoidance of mix-up.

4.26 Goods should be stored off the floor where possible, and in a manner that will permit easy cleaning and the use of pest-control agents (by trained personnel) without risk of contamination.

4.27 Generally, all goods should be stored under cover. Only goods whose conditions and labelling cannot be adversely affected by the weather should be stored out of doors.

4.28 All material containers should be clean before they are admitted to stores, and checked again for cleanliness before issue to manufacturing areas.

4.29 Where special storage conditions (eg temperature, humidity, security) are required, these should be provided, and checked and monitored. In particular, controlled temperature environments should be equipped with temperature recorders, combined with an automatic alarm, or with regular visual checking of the record. Corrective action should be taken as necessary.

Equipment

4.30 Equipment should be designed and located to suit the processes and products for which it is to be used. It should have been shown to be capable of carrying out the processes for which it is used, and of being operated to the necessary hygienic standards. It should be maintained so as to be fit to perform its functions and present no hazard to the product.

4.31 Manufacturing equipment should be easily and conveniently cleanable, both inside and out. There should be written instructions for such cleaning, and suitable cleaning facilities should be provided.

4.32 Equipment parts which come into contact with materials being processed should be minimally reactive or absorptive with respect to those materials.

4.33 Equipment should not hazard a product through leaking glands, lubricant drips, and the like; or through inappropriate modifications or adaptations.

4.34 Equipment should be kept or stored in a clean condition and be checked for cleanliness prior to each use.

4.35 Equipment should be sufficiently well spaced to avoid congestion and to ensure that products do not become admixed or confused with one another. (see also 5.13 and Appendix 2 on Cross Contamination).

4.36 Equipment used for weighing, measuring, testing and recording should be subject to regular recorded checks for accuracy and working order, according to a written planned maintenance schedule. Periodic comprehensive checks can usefully be supplemented by frequent simple checks on zero reading and accuracy.

4.37 Fixed pipework (and valves) should be clearly identified as to their contents.

5. MANUFACTURE

PRINCIPLES *Manufacture should follow previously defined procedures which are known to be capable of yielding finished products which are those intended and which conform to their specifications.*
Special attention must be paid to labels and labelling throughout the entire production cycle.

5.1 Production staff should follow defined and authorised procedures for each stage of each manufacturing process, ie the manufacture of a product should proceed in accordance with the Master Formula and Method, and/or with the Master Packaging Instruction (Ref 3.17 to 3.21), supplemented as necessary by Standard Operating Procedures. The details of the operation should be recorded on the Batch Manufacturing Record, or Batch Packaging Record (Ref 3.30 to 3.38).

5.2 Any deviation from defined procedures must be recorded and agreed by the person responsible for Production and the person responsible for Quality Control.

5.3 Before any manufacturing operation begins steps should be taken to ensure that the work area and equipment are clean and free from any starting material, packaging material, products, product-residues or documents not required for the current operation.

5.4 At all times during processing, all materials, bulk containers and major items of equipment used should be labelled or otherwise identified with an indication of the product or material being processed, its strength (where applicable) and batch number. Where applicable, this identification should also indicate the stage of manufacture and status.

5.5 Before applying labels or marks to materials or equipment, all inappropriate labels or marks previously applied should be removed or permanently defaced.

5.6 Containers and closures used for materials awaiting processing, for in-process products, and for bulk products, should be clean and of a nature and type which will prevent contamination or deterioration of the product or material.

5.7 The final yield, and any significant intermediate yield, of each production batch should be recorded and checked against the expected yield. In the event of a significant variation, steps should be taken to prevent release or further processing of the batch (or of any other batches, or products processed concurrently, with which it may have become admixed) until an adequate explanation can be found which permits release or further processing.

5.8 Further information on specific product types is given in Part II (Sections 9 to 13).

Validation

5.9 When any new Master Formula and Method is adopted steps should be taken to demonstrate that it is suitable for routine production and that the defined process, using the materials and equipment specified, will consistently yield a product of the required quality.

5.10 Significant changes in processing methods, equipment or materials should be accompanied by further validation steps to ensure that the changed conditions continue to yield consistently a product of the required quality.

5.11 From time to time processes and procedures should undergo critical appraisal to ensure that they remain capable of achieving the intended results.

5.12 Validation studies should be conducted in accordance with previously defined procedures and a record made of the results. The extent and degree of the work will depend on the nature and complexity of the product and process.

Contamination

5.13 The presence in a medicinal product of any chemical or microbiological contaminant, of such a nature and in such a quantity as may have the potential to affect adversely the health of any patient or impair the therapeutic activity of the product, is unacceptable. Particular attention should be paid to the problem of cross contamination, since even if it is of a nature and at a level unlikely to affect health directly, it may be indicative of unsatisfactory manufacturing practices. (For information on control of cross-contamination, see Appendix 2).

Starting Materials

5.14 Each starting material used should comply with its Starting Material Specification, and be labelled with the name designated in the specification before being released for use. Unauthorised abbreviations, codes or names should not be used.

5.15 Each delivery or batch of material should be assigned a reference number which will identify the delivery or batch throughout storage and processing. This number should appear on the container label(s) and permit access to records which will enable full details (including analytical reports) of the delivery to be checked. Different batches within one material delivery should be regarded as separate batches for sampling, testing and release purposes. (see 3.33 (a)).

5.16 Each delivery should be visually checked on receipt for general condition, integrity of container(s), spoilage and possible deterioration, and be sampled by personnel and methods approved by the person responsible for Quality Control. The samples should be tested for compliance with the starting material specification.

In certain circumstances, partial or entire compliance with specification may be demonstrated by the possession of a Certificate of Analysis, combined with first-hand assurance of identity (see Appendix 3 'Certificates of Analysis').

5.17 Care should be taken during sampling to guard against contamination of, or by, the material being sampled. All sampling equipment which comes in contact with the material must be clean. Some particularly hazardous or potent materials may require special precautions.

5.18 Steps should be taken to provide assurance that all containers in a delivery contain the correct starting material, and to safeguard against mislabelling of the containers by the supplier. (See Appendix 4 – 'Assurance of the Identity of Starting Materials').

5.19 Deliveries of Starting Materials should be held in quarantine (see Glossary) until released for use on the authority of the person responsible for Quality Control.

5.20 Status labels (see Glossary) should only be applied to Starting Materials by persons approved by the person responsible for Quality Control. Such labels should be of a nature or form which prevents confusion with any similar labels previously applied by the material supplier (eg they should be in a 'House Style' or bear the company name or logo). As the status of material changes, the status-labels should be changed accordingly (see also 5.4 and 5.5).

5.21 Stocks of Starting Materials should be inspected at intervals to ensure that the containers are properly closed and labelled, and in good condition. They should be re-sampled and submitted for re-test at the intervals given in the starting material specification. Such re-sampling should be initiated by the application of re-test date labels and/or by similarly effective documentary systems.

5.22 Materials should be issued for use only by authorised persons, following an approved and documented procedure. Stock records should be maintained so that stock reconciliations can be made.

5.23 Starting materials should only be dispensed by authorised persons, following a procedure defined in writing, to ensure that the correct materials are accurately weighed or measured into clean, properly labelled containers. Each dispensing operation should be checked independently and the check recorded. (See also 3.33 (f)).

5.24 Segregated dispensing areas, suitably equipped to avoid cross-contamination should be provided. Specially equipped 'dedicated' areas may be necessary for the dispensing of sensitising or highly toxic materials such as hormones, cytotoxic agents and certain antibiotics.

5.25 Weighing and measuring equipment should regularly be verified as accurate and should have the capacity, accuracy and precision appropriate to the amount of material to be weighed or measured.

Packaging Materials

5.26 The Packaging Materials used should comply with the relevant Packaging Material Specifications.

5.27 Each delivery or batch of Packaging Material should be awarded a reference number which will permit access to records which will enable full details (including test reports) of the delivery or batch to be checked.

5.28 Recording, checking, sampling and testing procedures should be followed for each delivery, in accordance with the Packaging Material Specification.

5.29 Printed Packaging Materials, and those which contact or may influence the product, should be held in quarantine until released for use on the authority of the person responsible for Quality Control. (See comments on status – labelling at 5.20).

5.30 Where possible, printed materials should bear identifying code numbers or marks as part of the printed text.

5.31 Packaging Materials should be issued for use only by an authorised person, using an approved and documented procedure. Stock records should be maintained so that stock reconciliations can be made.

[NOTE – Lesser standards of control and documentation may be applied to packaging materials which can have no influence on product quality – see note under 'Packaging Materials' in Glossary].

Intermediate Products

5.32 Each Intermediate Product which requires testing should be tested in accordance, and shown to comply, with its Specification. The records of such tests should be included in the batch documents.

5.33 Containers in which an Intermediate Product, partly packed product, or sub-batch is stored should be labelled or marked with an indication of product identity, quantity, batch and status.

Packaging

5.34 All packaging operations should proceed in accordance with the instructions given, and using the materials specified, in the Master Packaging Instruction (Ref. 3.21), supplemented as necessary by Standard Operating Procedures. Details of the operation should be recorded on the Batch Packaging Record (Ref. 3.34 – 3.38).

5.35 Before a packaging operation begins, checks should be made to ensure that the work area and equipment are clean and free from any product, product residues, materials, labels or documents not required for that operation. The record of these checks should form part of the batch packaging documentation. (Ref. 3.36).

5.36 Products of similar appearance should not be packaged in close proximity unless there is physical segregation.

5.37 At each packaging station or line the name and batch of the product being handled should be prominently displayed.

5.38 *All possible steps should be taken to avoid labelling and packaging errors.* (For appropriate measures, see Appendix 5).

5.39 Containers to be filled should be supplied to the packaging line or station in a clean condition, or be cleaned on-line.

5.40 On completion of a packaging operation, any unused batch-coded labels and materials should be destroyed. A documented standard procedure should be used if any uncoded materials are returned to stock. (See also 3.38).

5.41 Packed Finished Products should be quarantined until released by Quality Control.

5.42 Measures should be taken to control the spread of dust during packaging of dry products, and to control airborne contamination during packaging of all products. Segregated packaging areas are necessary for some products (eg potent low-dose or toxic products and sensitising agents).

5.43 Products filled into their final containers and held awaiting labelling should be segregated and marked so as to avoid mix-ups.

Finished Product Release

5.44 A finished product should only be passed into usable stock (ie stock which may be distributed, sold or supplied for use) after it has been formally released on the authority of the person responsible for Quality Control. Finished product evaluation should embrace all relevant factors, including manufacturing conditions, results of in-process testing, a review of manufacturing (including packaging) documentation, compliance with Finished Product Specification and examination of the final finished pack.

Any unexplained yield discrepancies or failures to comply with specifications should be thoroughly investigated, with consideration extended to other batches or other products which might also be affected.

Storage

5.45 Materials and products should be stored under conditions which minimise deterioration, contamination, spillage or breakage.

5.46 Special attention should be given to the security of all stored labels and other printed packaging materials. Cut labels and other loose printed packaging materials should be stored in closed containers.

5.47 Where special environmental conditions are required for certain materials and products, these conditions should be continuously monitored, and corrective action taken where necessary.

5.48 Materials and products should be stored in an orderly fashion to avoid confusion, to allow batch differentiation and rotation of stocks, and to permit easy cleaning.

5.49 Storage arrangements should allow pest control materials to be effectively employed by trained personnel, whilst avoiding contamination of materials or products.

5.50 If sampling in stores is appropriate for the materials handled, provision should be made for it to be done effectively, without the risk of contamination from other materials or the environment, or of other materials by the material being sampled.

5.51 Where a separate quarantine area is provided, access should be restricted to authorised persons.

5.52 Great care should be taken to ensure that goods which have been rejected, recalled or returned are suitably labelled and segregated to avoid confusion with other materials and products.

5.53 Stores should be regularly checked for cleanliness and good order and for misplaced, deteriorated, or out-dated stock.

Transport and Distribution

5.54 Materials and Finished Products should be transported both inside and outside the factory by means which ensure that:

(a) Product identification is not lost.

(b) No confusion arises between a consignment which is suitable for use, and other consignments of the same product or materials which are not.

(c) A product does not contaminate, and is not contaminated by, other products or materials.

(d) Adequate precautions are taken against spillage or breakage.

(e) A product and its pack are not damaged by heat, cold, light, moisture or attack by micro-organisms or pests, or by other adverse influences.

5.55 Labels and other printed packaging materials should be transported (eg from stores to packaging line) in a secure manner. If they are not for immediate use, they should be held securely in the packaging area.

6. RECOVERED MATERIALS

PRINCIPLE

Material may be re-worked or recovered by an appropriate and authorised method, provided that the material is suitable for such reprocessing, that the resultant product meets its specification and there are no significant changes in product quality. Documentation should accurately record the reworking processes carried out.

Product Residues

6.1 Residues and re-worked or recovered material which might adversely affect product quality, efficacy or safety should not be used in subsequent batches.

6.2 The treatment of product residues and reworked or recovered material and the means of their inclusion in a subsequent batch should be specifically authorised and documented.

6.3 Limits, approved by Quality Control, should be established for the amount of any such material which may be added to a subsequent batch.

6.4 Batches incorporating residues should not be released until the batches from which the residues originated have been tested and found suitable for use.

Re-processing

6.5 Methods of re-processing should be specifically authorised and fully documented, once any potential risks have been evaluated and found negligible.

6.6 The need for additional testing of any Finished Product which has been re-processed (or to which residues have been added) should be considered.

Returned Goods

6.7 A Finished Product returned from the Manufacturer's own stores or warehouse (because, for example, of soiled or damaged labels or outer packaging) may be relabelled or bulked for inclusion in subsequent batches, provided that there is no risk to product quality and the operation is specifically authorised and documented. If such products are re-labelled, extra care is necessary to avoid mix-up or mis-labelling.

6.8 Finished Products returned from the market and which have left the control of the manufacturer should be considered for re-sale, re-labelling or bulking with a subsequent batch only after they have been critically assessed by the person responsible for Quality Control. The nature of the product, any special storage conditions it requires, its condition and history, and the time elapsed since it was issued should all be taken into account in this assessment. Where any doubt arises over the quality of the product, it should not be considered suitable for re-issue or re-use, although basic chemical re-processing to recover active ingredient may be possible.

7. COMPLAINTS PROCEDURES AND PRODUCT RECALL

PRINCIPLE

The full significance of a complaint may only be appreciated by certain responsible persons, and then possibly only with the knowledge of other related complaints. A procedure must therefore exist to channel complaint reports appropriately.

A complaint, or otherwise reported product-defect, may lead to the need for a recall. Any action taken to recall a product suspected or known to be defective or hazardous, should be prompt and in accordance with a pre-determined plan. The procedures to be followed should be specified in writing and made known to all who may be concerned.

Complaints

7.1 A system should be established for dealing with complaints which should include written procedures indicating the responsible person(s) through whom the complaints are to be channelled. The responsible person must have appropriate knowledge and experience and the necessary authority to decide the action to be taken.

7.2 All complaints concerning product quality must be thoroughly investigated. The responsible person should decide whether, and what, subsequent action is necessary. This action should be recorded and the record filed with the details of the original complaint. (See also under 'Documentation' 3.42).

7.3 Complaint records should be regularly reviewed for any indication of a need for recall or of specific problems requiring attention.

Recall Procedure

7.4 A responsible person (or persons) with suitable deputies should be nominated to initiate and co-ordinate all recall activities.

7.5 There should be a written recall procedure which is capable of being put into operation at any time, inside or outside normal working hours. It should include emergency and 'out of hours' contacts and telephone numbers. Records of distribution should be kept which will facilitate effective recall.

7.6 The recall procedure should be shown to be practicable and operable within reasonable time (eg by conducting internal 'dummy runs'). It should be revised as necessary to take account of changes in procedures or responsible person(s).

7.7 The procedure should indicate:

(a) The methods to be used for halting the distribution of the batch or batches which are the subject of an adverse report.

(b) The means of consultation with the Defect Report Centre of Medicines Division of the Department of Health and Social Security and the circumstances in which this is needed. (In critical situations involving a risk to patients, such consultation is essential).

(c) The means of notifying and implementing a recall, and of deciding its extent.

7.8 The notification of recall should include:

(a) The name of the product, its strength and pack size.

(b) The product batch number(s).

(c) The nature of the defect.

(d) The action to be taken.

(e) The urgency of the action (with reasons, indication of health risk, as appropriate).

7.9 Account should be taken of any goods which may be in transit when the recall is initiated.

7.10 The progress and efficacy of a recall should be assessed at intervals.

7.11 Any recalled products should be placed immediately in quarantine.

7.12 When a defective product is discovered or suspected the possibility that the fault may extend to other batches or to other products (eg through the use of a faulty or incorrect material in several batches of product, or through a fault in a widely used piece of equipment) should be considered and appropriate action taken.

8. GOOD CONTROL LABORATORY PRACTICE

PRINCIPLE

It is essential that control laboratories should have appropriate facilities, with properly trained, managed and motivated staff, in order that reliable results may be obtained from any analytical or other test procedure, whether its nature is chemical, physical, biological or microbiological. Steps should be taken to ensure the reliability of the laboratory's own systems and test methods.

[NOTE – This section provides additional guidelines for good laboratory practice to be applied in pharmaceutical control laboratories. Where relevant, principles outlined elsewhere in this Guide apply. (See especially the sections on 'Personnel and Training', and on 'Documentation'). Additional measures may be necessary in specialised control laboratories, e.g. laboratories handling radioactive or biological samples.]

Premises

8.1 Control laboratories should be designed, equipped, maintained and of sufficient space to suit the operations to be performed in them, and include provision for writing and recording and the storage of documents and samples.

8.2 Chemical, biological and microbiological laboratories should be separated from each other and from manufacturing areas. Separate rooms may be necessary to protect sensitive instruments from vibration, electrical interference, humidity etc.

8.3 Provision should be made for the safe storage of waste materials awaiting disposal.

8.4 All services should be marked with an indication of identity.

Equipment

8.5 Control laboratory equipment and instrumentation should be appropriate to the testing procedures undertaken.

8.6 Equipment and instruments should be serviced and calibrated at suitable specified intervals by an assigned person, persons, or organisation, and readily available records maintained for each instrument or piece of equipment. These records should indicate when the next calibration or servicing is due.

8.7 Written operating instructions should be readily available for each instrument.

8.8 Where practicable, suitable arrangements should be made to indicate failure of equipment or services to equipment. Defective equipment should be withdrawn from use until the fault has been rectified.

8.9 As necessary, analytical methods should include a step to verify that the equipment is functioning satisfactorily.

Cleanliness

8.10 Control laboratories and equipment should be kept clean, in accordance with written cleaning schedules.

8.11 Personnel should wear clean protective clothing appropriate to the duties being performed.

8.12 The disposal of waste material should be carefully and responsibly undertaken.

Reagents etc

8.13 Where necessary reagents should be dated upon receipt or preparation.

8.14 Reagents made up in the laboratory should be prepared by persons competent to do so, following laid-down procedures. As applicable labelling should indicate the concentration, standardisation factor, shelf life, and storage conditions. The label should be initialled or signed, and dated, by the person preparing the reagent. As relevant a date for re-standardisation should be recorded.

8.15 In certain cases, it may be necessary to carry out tests to confirm that the reagent is suitable for the purpose for which it is to be used. A record of these tests should be maintained.

8.16 Both positive and negative controls should be applied to verify the suitability of microbiological culture media. The size of the inoculum used in positive controls should be appropriate to the sensitivity required.

8.17 Reference standards, and any secondary standards prepared from them, should be dated and be stored, handled and used so as not to prejudice their quality.

Sampling

8.18 Samples should be taken in such a manner that they are representative of the batches of material from which they are taken, in accordance with written sampling procedures approved by the person responsible for Quality Control. These procedures should include:

(i) The method of sampling.
(ii) The equipment to be used.
(iii) The amount of sample to be taken.
(iv) Instructions for any required sub-division of the sample.
(v) The type and condition of sample container to be used.
(vi) Any special precautions to be observed, especially in regard to sampling of sterile or noxious materials.
(vii) Cleaning and storage of sampling equipment.

Any sampling by production personnel should only be done in accordance with these approved procedures.

8.19 Each sample container should bear a label indicating its contents, with the batch or lot number reference and the date of sampling. It should also be possible to identify the bulk containers from which samples have been drawn.

8.20 Sampling equipment should be cleaned after each use and stored separately from other laboratory equipment.

8.21 Care should be taken to avoid contamination, or causing deterioration, whenever a material or product is sampled. Special care is necessary when re-sealing sampled containers to prevent damage to, or contamination of, or by, the contents.

Documentation

8.22 Laboratory documentation should be in line with the general guidance given in the section on 'Documentation' (ref 3.1 to 3.6). When electronic or magnetic methods are used, see also section on Electronic Data Processing. (Section 16).

8.23 Retention samples should be regarded as part of the laboratory records.

8.24 It is useful to record test results in a manner that will facilitate comparative reviews of those results and the detection of trends.

Records of Analysis

8.25 Details to be recorded on the receipt and testing of Starting Materials, Packaging Materials and Intermediate, Bulk and Finished Products are given at 3.22, 3.23, 3.26, 3.27, 3.29 and 3.39. For ease of reference a summary of analytical record requirements is given here, as follows. These records should contain:

- (i) Name of product or material and code reference.
- (ii) Date of receipt and sampling.
- (iii) Source of product or material.
- (iv) Date of testing.
- (v) Batch or Lot number.
- (vi) Indication of tests performed.
- (vii) Reference to the method used.
- (viii) Results.
- (ix) Decision regarding release, rejection or other status.
- (x) Signature or initials of analyst, and signature of person taking the above decision.

8.26 In addition to the above records, analysts' laboratory records should also be retained, with the basic data and calculations from which test results were derived (e.g. weighings, readings, recorder charts etc).

[NOTE – For information on retention of Reference Samples see 3.25, 3.40 and 3.43].

Specifications

8.27 Specifications approved by Quality Control should be established for all starting materials, packaging materials and Bulk, Intermediate and Finished Products. Details of these specifications are given in the section on Documentation (ref 3.8 to 3.15).

Testing

8.28 The persons responsible for laboratory management should ensure that suitable test-methods, validated in the context of available facilities and equipment, are adopted or developed.

8.29 Samples should be tested in accordance with the test-methods referred to, or detailed, in the relevant specifications. The validity of the results obtained should be checked (and as necessary, any calculations checked) before the material is released or rejected.

8.30 In-process control work carried out by production staff should proceed in accordance with methods approved by the person responsible for Quality Control.

Contract Analysis

8.31 Although analysis and testing may be undertaken by a Contract Analyst, the responsibility for Quality Control *cannot* be delegated to him.

8.32 The nature and extent of any contract analysis to be undertaken should be agreed and clearly defined in writing, and procedures for taking samples should be as set out abcve. (8.18–8.21).

8.33 The Contract Analyst should be supplied with full details of the test methods relevant to the material under examination. These will need to be confirmed as suitable for use in the context of the contract laboratory.

8.34 Formal arrangements should be made for the retention of samples and of records of test results.

[NOTE – See also section 14 'Contract Manufacture, Analysis and Servicing'].

Part Two

9. MANUFACTURE AND CONTROL OF STERILE MEDICINAL PRODUCTS

PRINCIPLES

Sterile products should be manufactured with special care and attention to detail, with the object of eliminating microbial and particulate contamination. Much depends on the skill, training and attitudes of the personnel involved. Even more than with other types of medicinal product, it is not sufficient that the finished product passes the specified tests, and in-process Quality Assurance assumes a singular importance.

General Considerations

9.1 Sterile products may be classified broadly into two categories, according to their manner of production; those which must be processed by aseptic means at some or all stages, and those which are sterilised when sealed in their final container ('terminally sterilised'). Whenever possible, sterile products should be terminally sterilised.

9.2 All sterile products should be manufactured under carefully controlled and monitored conditions, and sole reliance should NOT be placed on any terminal process or test for assurance of the microbial and particulate quality of the end-product.

9.3 To provide assurance of sterility, special precautions are necessary in the aseptic processing of products which are not subject to terminal sterilisation.

Definitions

9.4 The following definitions, some of which are additional to those given in the Glossary, are especially significant in the context of sterile production.

Air Lock: An enclosed space, with two or more doors only one of which should normally be capable of being opened at any one time, and which is interposed between two or more rooms (e.g. of differing classes of cleanliness) to control the air-flow between those rooms when they need to be entered. An air lock may be designed for and used by either personnel or materials.

Aseptic Area: A room, suite of rooms or special area within a Clean Area (see below) designed, constructed, serviced and used with the intention of preventing microbial contamination of the product.

Batch: As defined in the Glossary, with the further proviso that for the purpose of a sterility test, a batch is a collection of sealed containers prepared in such a manner that the risk of microbial contamination may be considered the same for each of the units in it. It is usually:

(a) one steriliser load, or

(b) the quantity of containers filled aseptically in one working session at one work station.

(In the case of aseptically filled products which are subsequently freeze-dried it should be one freeze-drier load if this is less than in (b) above). A working session should be deemed to terminate whenever there is a significant change in circumstances which could affect the risk of product contamination (for example, a change of filling equipment, a change in the team of operators or a machine break-down). What in fact constitutes 'a significant change' should be documented and agreed in advance by the persons responsible for Production and Quality Control.

Changing Room: A room or suite of rooms designed for the changing of clothes and from which a clean or aseptic area is entered.

Clean Area: A room or suite of rooms with defined environmental control of particulate and microbial contamination, constructed and used in such a way as to reduce the introduction, generation and retention of contaminants within the area.

Contained Work Station: A small working area or enclosure with its own, usually unidirectional, filtered air supply.

Monitor: – See Glossary.

Sterlity (etc): – See Glossary.

Basic Environmental Standards: Aseptic Areas

9.5 For aseptic processing, rooms with conventional filtered air-flows and with contained work stations in the form of filtered-air hoods or laminar air flow protection at working points are usually more appropriate than laminar air flow rooms.

9.6 Rooms for aseptic processing should, in the unmanned state, comply with the conditions specified for Grade 1/B in the Table of

Basic Environmental Standards (Appendix 1). With people present and work in progress, Grade 1/A (Appendix 1) conditions should be maintained under the contained work stations where products are exposed and aseptic manipulations carried-out.

Basic Environmental Standards: Clean Areas for Solution Preparation

9.7 Solutions intended for use as large or small volume parenterals, eye-drops, contact lens solutions, peritoneal dialysis solutions, and for irrigation (including non-intravenous water for irrigation use) should be prepared in a room complying with the conditions specified for Grade 2 in Appendix 1. The object should be to prepare a pyrogen-free solution with low microbial and particulate counts, suitable for later sterilisation.

Products such as suspensions, ointments and creams which are to be terminally sterilised should also be prepared under Grade 2 conditions.

[NOTE – When powders for solution or suspension etc are being handled a temporarily lower *particulate* standard may in consequence be inevitable].

9.8 As an alternative it may be possible to prepare solutions in a room of Grade 3 (Appendix 1) standard, provided additional steps are taken to achieve the objectives outlined in 9.7 above. Thus the solution could be sterile-filtered via a closed system immediately following preparation, and then either collected in a clean, sterilised, sealed vessel (with any outlets sealed by sterilising grade filters), or filled directly into final containers and terminally sterilised within a specified short time.

Basic Environmental Standards: Clean Rooms for Filling Solutions etc

9.9 The filling of products to be terminally sterilised should be carried out in rooms complying with the conditions specified for Grade 2 (Appendix 1). Extra precautions in the form of contained work stations and/or laminar air flow protection, are necessary when solutions intended for intravenous use are filled into wide-necked containers.

Basic Environmental Standards: Clean Areas for Component Preparation

9.10 Special environmental standards may not be necessary for areas used for the *initial* preparation of such packaging components as ampoules, vials, bottles, closures, and droppers, but appropriate care should be taken throughout to ensure that they are clean (and, as necessary, sterile) and do not endanger the microbial or particulate quality of the product. Following the final cleaning process they should be handled in such an environment and manner as will prevent recontamination.

Basic Environmental Standards: Microbiological Considerations

9.11 It is vital that microbial contamination of clean and aseptic areas should not exceed acceptable limits. Such areas should be monitored for microbial contamination by such methods as 'settle' plates, air samplers and surface swabs etc.

9.12 In a new unit, with a new process or with new operators microbial monitoring should be sufficiently intensive to determine patterns and levels of contamination. Once suitable conditions have been established, monitoring may be reduced to a level which will demonstrate maintenance of those conditions. (See also 9.41 to 9.43).

Personnel

9.13 Personnel required to work in clean and aseptic areas should be selected with care to ensure that they may be relied upon to observe the appropriate disciplines and are not subject to any disease or condition which would present an abnormal microbiological hazard to the product.

9.14 High standards of personal hygiene and cleanliness are essential. Staff should be instructed to report any condition (e.g. diarrhoea, coughs, colds, infected skin or hair, wounds etc) which may cause the shedding of abnormal numbers or types of organisms. Periodic health checks for such conditions are desirable.

9.15 Only the minimum required number of personnel should be present in clean and aseptic areas when work is in progress. Inspection and control procedures should be conducted from outside the areas as far as possible.

9.16 All personnel (including those concerned with maintenance) employed in such areas should receive training in the disciplines relevant to the successful manufacture of sterile products, including reference to hygiene and at least the basic elements of microbiology. Initial training should be followed by suitable refresher courses.

9.17 When outside staff who have not received such training (e.g. building or maintenance contractors) need to be brought in, particular care should be taken over their supervision. They should be appropriately dressed (see below).

9.18 Staff who have been engaged in the processing of animal tissue materials or of cultures of micro-organisms other than those used in the current manufacturing process should not enter sterile-product areas unless rigorous and clearly defined decontamination procedures have been followed.

Clothing

9.19 Operators and their garments are, potentially, the most significant sources of microbial and particulate contamination. Personnel entering clean or aseptic areas should change into special garments which includes head and foot wear. These garments should shed virtually no fibres or particulate matter, and retain particles shed by the body. They should be comfortable to wear, and loose fitting to reduce abrasion. Fabric edges should be sealed and seams all-enveloping. Unnecessary tucks or belts should be avoided, and there should be no external pockets. The garments should be restricted to use only in the relevant clean or aseptic areas.

9.20 In aseptic areas personnel should wear sterilised single or two-piece trouser-suits, gathered at the wrists and ankles and with high necks. Headgear must totally enclose hair and beard and be of the helmet/cowl type, tucked into the neck of the suit. Footwear should totally enclose the feet, and trouser-bottoms should be tucked inside the foot-wear.

Fresh clean and sterilised protective garments should normally be provided each time a person enters an aseptic area. Powder-free rubber or plastic gloves should be worn with the garment sleeves tucked inside the gloves. A non-linting face mask should also be worn. It should be comfortable to wear, and prevent the shedding of droplets. It should be discarded at least each time the aseptic area is left.

9.21 Outdoor clothing should not be brought into the changing rooms associated with clean or aseptic areas, and personnel entering these changing rooms should already be clad in standard factory protective garments. Changing and washing should follow a clearly displayed written procedure.

9.22 Bulky or fluffy personal clothing should be removed before aseptic or clean room garments are donned. Wristwatches and jewellery other than a simple wedding ring should not be worn. Cosmetics which can shed particles should not be used.

9.23 Clean and aseptic area clothing should be laundered or cleaned and thereafter handled in such a way that it does not gather contaminants which can later be shed. Separate laundry facilities for such clothing are desirable. It should be noted that some methods of sterilisation may damage fibres and reduce effective garment life.

Premises

9.24 Sterile medicinal products should be prepared in specially designed and constructed manufacturing departments which are separate from other manufacturing areas, and in which the different types of operation such as component preparation, solution preparation, filling and sterilisation are effectively segregated one from another.

9.25 The various processing rooms should be supplied and effectively flushed with air under positive pressure, which has passed through filters of appropriate designated efficiency and which will maintain a positive pressure differential relative to surrounding areas (and as necessary *between* different areas within a suite of rooms) under all operational conditions. Final air filtration should be at or as close as possible to the point of input to a room. A warning system should indicate failure in the air supply, and an indicator of pressure differential should be fitted between areas where this differential is critical. Particular attention should be given to the zone of greatest risk, that is, the immediate environment to which a product is exposed. (see 9.5–9.11, and Appendix 1). Where contained work stations are employed, care should be taken to ensure that air flows do not distribute particles from a particle-generating person, operation, or machine (ampoule cutter, capper etc) to a zone of higher product risk.

[NOTE – The various recommendations regarding air supplies and pressure differentials may need to be modified where it becomes necessary to contain pathogenic, highly toxic or radioactive materials. In such circumstances microbiological safety cabinets complying with BS 5726 should be used. Cabinets giving horizontal air-flow should NOT be used].

9.26 Non-sterile products should not be processed in the same area and at the same time as sterile products. If non-sterile procedures are carried out in rooms normally designated as aseptic these rooms must be suitably disinfected, flushed with filtered air, and verified as conforming to the required standard before reverting to sterile production.

9.27 Vaccines of dead organisms, or of bacterial extracts, may be filled (after inactivation) in the same premises as other sterile medicinal products. Spore forming organisms should be processed in separate premises or well isolated suites at least until any inactivation stage is completed. Live or attenuated vaccines should be processed and filled in premises separate from other processing or filling operations. Different live vaccines should be processed and filled separately from each other. Separation may be achieved in space or, given adequate cleaning and disinfection, in time. Special isolation facilities may be needed for highly contagious micro-organisms.

9.28 The processing of animal tissue materials and of micro-organisms not required for the current manufacturing process, the performance of test procedures involving animals or micro-organisms, and any animal houses must be well separated from premises for manufacturing sterile medicinal products, with completely separate ventilation systems, and separate staff.

9.29 The surfaces of walls, floors and ceilings should be smooth, impervious and unbroken in order to minimise the shedding or accumulation of particulate matter, and to permit the repeated application of cleaning agents and disinfectants where used. Bare wood should be avoided.

9.30 To reduce accumulation of dust and to facilitate cleaning, there should be no uncleanable recesses and a minimum of projecting ledges, shelves, cupboards, equipment, fixtures and fittings. Coving should be used where walls meet floors and ceilings in aseptic areas (and preferably in other clean areas as well). Care should be taken to ensure that the coving is installed so as not to create additional dust-accumulating ridges.

9.31 False ceilings should be adequately sealed to prevent contamination from the space above them.

9.32 Pipes and ducts should be installed so that they do not create recesses which are difficult to clean. They should be sealed into walls through which they pass.

9.33 Drains should be avoided wherever possible, and excluded from aseptic areas unless essential. Where installed they should be fitted with effective, easily cleanable traps and with air breaks to prevent back-flow. The traps may contain electrically operated heating devices or other means for disinfection. Any floor channels should be open, shallow and easily cleanable and be connected to drains outside the area in a manner which prevents ingress of microbial contaminants.

9.34 Sinks should be excluded from aseptic areas. Any sinks installed in other clean areas should be of stainless steel, without overflow, and be supplied with water of at least potable quality.

9.35 Room temperature and humidity should be maintained at a level which will not cause excessive sweating of operators clad in protective garments.

9.36 Access to clean and aseptic areas should be restricted to authorised persons, who enter only through changing rooms where normal factory clothing is exchanged for special protective garments. (See 9.19 to 9.23). Changing rooms should be air-locked and effectively flushed with filtered air at a positive pressure lower than that in the clean and aseptic processing rooms. They should be designed and used so as to minimise microbial and particulate contamination of protective garments, and to provide separation of the different stages of changing and, as necessary, washing. A written changing procedure should be followed.

9.37 Under routine operating conditions changing rooms should be for personnel only, and should not normally be used for the passage of materials, containers and equipment.

9.38 Hatchways and airlocks for the passage of materials, equipment and other goods into clean and aseptic areas should be arranged so that only one side may be opened at any one time. Because of difficulties in cleaning the sliding gear, sliding doors should be avoided. Conveyor belts should not pass through walls enclosing aseptic areas. They should end at the wall, products passing onwards across a stationary surface. Special precautions are necessary to avoid contamination of aseptic areas when articles are passed through air-locks or hatchways.

9.39 Electrical/mechanical systems for oral communication from and to aseptic areas should be designed and installed so that they may be effectively cleaned and disinfected.

9.40 Clean and aseptic processing areas should not be used for sterility, or other microbiological, test procedures.

Cleanliness and Hygiene

9.41 Clean, aseptic and other related processing areas should be cleaned frequently and thoroughly in accordance with a written programme approved by the Quality Control Department. Where disinfectants are used, different types should be employed in rotation to discourage the development of resistant strains of micro-organisms.

9.42 Disinfectants and detergents used should be monitored for microbial contamination. Dilutions should be kept in previously cleaned containers and should not be stored unless sterilised. Partly emptied containers should not be refilled.

9.43 Areas should be frequently monitored microbiologically by means of 'settle' plates, surface sampling, air sampling or other appropriate methods. The monitoring should be performed whilst normal production operations are in progress. Records should be retained and immediate remedial action taken as soon as results deviate significantly from those usually found in the area concerned. (See 9.11 and 9.12).

Equipment

9.44 Equipment should be designed and installed so that it may be easily cleaned, disinfected or sterilised as required.

9.45 As far as possible equipment fittings and services should be designed and installed so that maintenance and repairs may be carried out without additional personnel having to enter the clean or aseptic rooms. If maintenance must be carried out within these areas, personnel concerned should receive appropriate training in the elements of microbiology and sterile area procedures. When within the areas they should be appropriately dressed, and use tools and equipment which have been sterilised or disinfected. Areas entered for maintenance should be cleaned and disinfected before processing recommences if the required standards of cleanliness or asepsis have not been maintained during the work.

9.46 Recording apparatus should be accurately calibrated on installation and thereafter checked at scheduled intervals.

9.47 Validation of performance on installation, planned maintenance, and frequent checks on performance are essential for critical items of equipment such as sterilisers, air filtration systems, and stills. For example, checks on steam and hot air sterilisers should include heat distribution and heat penetration studies, and on air supply systems, tests of filter efficiency. (See Health Technical Memorandum No 10, 'Sterilisers', HMSO 1980, and BS 5295). Details of maintenance operations and performance checks should be recorded.

Processing

9.48 Starting materials should not contain significant levels of microorganisms or pyrogenic material. The material specifications should include requirements for microbiological monitoring, with limits as necessary.

9.49 Precautions should be taken during all processing stages before and after sterilisation to avoid contamination of the product with micro-organisms.

9.50 Activities in clean and aseptic areas should be kept to a minimum. Movements of personnel should be controlled and methodical, to avoid excessive shedding of particles and organisms due to over-vigorous activity.

9.51 Containers and other materials liable to generate particles or fibres should not be taken into clean or aseptic areas.

9.52 Components and containers should be handled after the final cleaning process in such a way that they are not subject to recontamination. The final rinse should be with purified water of appropriate quality.

9.53 The interval between the washing and the subsequent sterilisation of equipment, containers and components should be kept to a minimum.

9.54 The interval between the sterilisation of equipment, containers and components, and their use in an aseptic process, should be kept to a minimum.

9.55 The interval between commencing preparation of a solution and its sterilisation should be kept to a minimum. This interval should be subject to a defined time-limit. Unless special storage precautions are taken, bulk solutions should have no greater volume than can be filled in one day and should be filled into final containers and sterilised within one working day.

9.56 Water treatment plants should be designed, constructed, and maintained to ensure the reliable production of water of the required quality. They should not be operated beyond their designed capacity. The water should be produced, stored and distributed in such a manner as to discourage microbial growth (e.g., by constant circulation at temperatures above 65°C, and avoidance of places where water may remain stagnant such as U-bends, 'dead ends' and ill-designed valves).

9.57 Water sources, water treatment equipment and treated water should be monitored regularly for chemical, microbial and pyrogen contamination as relevant. Records should be maintained of the results of the monitoring, and of any remedial action.

9.58 Unsterilised distilled water intended for further processing or sterilisation should not stand for more than a short time unless special precautions are taken, such as storage above 65°C, to prevent both the growth of bacteria and the consequent development of pyrogens.

9.59 Where water or solutions are held in sealed vessels, any pressure relief outlets should be protected by hydrophobic microbial air filters.

9.60 Articles required in an aseptic area should be sterilised and passed into the area through double-ended sterilisers sealed into the wall, or by other methods which will achieve the same end of avoiding contamination of the area or the articles.

9.61 When a new aseptic process is introduced, when any significant change is made in such a process or in the equipment, when staff are being trained and at regular intervals thereafter, the efficacy of aseptic procedures should be validated, e.g. by filling a sterile liquid nutrient medium or powder and testing for the incidence of contamination. Such fillings should be carried out under normal operating conditions.

Sterilisation
General

9.62 Sterilisation can be effected by moist or dry heat, by ethylene oxide (or other suitable gaseous sterilant), by filtration with subsequent aseptic filling into sterile final containers, or by irradiation with ionizing radiations (but not with untraviolet radiation). Each method has its particular applications and limitations. Where possible and practicable heat sterilisation is the method of choice.

9.63 For effective sterilisation, the whole of the material must be subjected to the required treatment, and the process must be designed and monitored to ensure that this is achieved.

9.64 Before any sterilisation process is adopted its suitability for the product and its efficacy in achieving the desired sterilising conditions in all parts of each type of load to be processed should be confirmed. Such validation should be repeated at suitable scheduled intervals and whenever significant modifications have been made to the equipment. Records should be kept of the results.

9.65 Materials and products to be sterilised should not carry a high level of microbial contamination. There should be a limit on microbial contamination immediately before sterilisation which is related to the efficiency of the method to be used. Large volume infusion fluids, in particular, should be passed through a bacteria-retaining filter before filling and sterilisation. The microbial contamination levels of products prior to sterilisation should be monitored, irrespective of the method of sterilisation employed.

9.66 If biological indicators are used, strict precautions should be taken to avoid transferring microbial contamination from them. (See 9.106 et seq).

9.67 There should be a clear means of differentiating products which have not been sterilised from those which have. Each basket, tray or other carrier of products or components should be clearly labelled with the material name, its batch number and an indication of whether or not it has been sterilised. Indicators such as autoclave tape may be used, where appropriate, to indicate whether or not a lot (or sub-lot) has passed through a sterilisation process, but they do not give a reliable indication that the lot is, in fact, sterile.

Heat Sterilisation: General

9.68 Each heat sterilisation cycle should be recorded on a temperature-time chart or by other suitable automatic means. If the former is used the scale should be large enough to permit reading of both time and temperature. The temperature should be measured from a probe at the coolest part of the loaded chamber, this point having been previously determined for each type of load to be processed. (In steam sterilisers with a chamber drain this point will commonly be at the drain itself). The time/temperature record should form part of the batch record. Where control of the sterilising cycle is automatic the heat-sensing control probe should be independent of the recording probe. Chemical or biological indicators may be used in addition, but should not take the place of physical controls.

9.69 After the high temperature phase of a heat sterilisation cycle, precautions should be taken against contamination of a sterilised load during cooling. Unless it can be shown that the product cannot be contaminated by it, any cooling fluid should be sterile. Precautions should be taken to prevent contamination by non-sterile air entering the autoclave or oven as it cools.

Heat Sterilisation: Moist Heat

9.70 [NOTE – This method is suitable only for water – wettable materials and aqueous solutions. Other materials must be sterilised by other methods].

Moist heat sterilisation is achieved by exposure to saturated steam under pressure in a suitably designed chamber (see BS 3970). In these circumstances there is an exact relationship between steam temperature and pressure, but the pressure is used solely to obtain the temperature required and otherwise contributes nothing to the sterilisation process. The temperature and *not* the pressure must be used to control and monitor the process.

9.71 Whilst temperatures and periods of treatment are recommended in official compendia, (e.g. 121°C for 15 minutes), other combinations of temperature and time can be used provided they have been validated. It is important to recognise that the temperature–time relationship is complex, that at temperatures below 115°C disproportionately long periods of time are required, and that as temperature is reduced the process may become progressively less reliable.

9.72 Items to be sterilised (other than aqueous medicinal products in sealed containers) should be wrapped in a material which allows removal of air and penetration of steam, and which under normal conditions does not permit recontamination by micro-organisms after sterilisation.

9.73 Unless special precautions are taken (see 9.74 below) air must be displaced from the chamber, and from materials within the chamber, either by a period of free steaming before the sterilisation cycle begins or by use of a vacuum pump.

9.74 Mixtures of steam with air may be used for sterilising sealed containers of aqueous fluids provided that steps are taken to ensure homogeneity of the steam-air mixture throughout the chamber, and the process has been validated.

9.75 Sufficient time must be allowed for the whole of the load to reach the required temperature before measurement of the sterilising time-period is commenced. This time must be determined for each type of load to be processed before the method is adopted.

9.76 Care should be taken to ensure that steam used for sterilisation is of suitable quality and does not contain additives at a level which could cause contamination of product or equipment.

Heat Sterilisation: Dry Heat

9.77 Dry heat is suitable for sterilising equipment, non-aqueous liquids and other materials which can withstand the temperatures required. Various combinations of temperature and time are recommended in official compendia but other combinations of temperature and time can be used provided they have been validated.

9.78 Heating should be carried out in an oven or other equipment which will achieve sterilising conditions throughout the load. (See BS 3421: Performance of Electrically-heated Sterilising Ovens). The method of loading used should not be such as to lead to an uneven temperature distribution.

9.79 Before the timed sterilisation period begins, sufficient time must be allowed for the temperature of the whole load to reach the requisite level. This time should be determined for each type of load to be processed, and the timed sterilisation period should not start until the entire load is known to have reached that level.

Sterilisation: Filtration

9.80 Sterilisation by filtration should not be used when sterilisation by heat is practicable.

9.81 Solutions or liquids can be sterilised by filtration through a sterile filter of nominal pore size of 0.22 micron (or less), or with at least equivalent micro-organism retaining properties, into a previously sterilised container. Such filters can remove bacteria and moulds but not all viruses or mycoplasmas.

9.82 The integrity of the filter assembly should be checked by an appropriate method, such as a bubble-point pressure test or forward-flow pressure test immediately before and after use. Abnormal filtration flow-rates should be noted and investigated. Results of these filter-integrity checks should be recorded in the batch record.

9.83 Filters containing asbestos should not be used. Any potentially fibre or particle releasing filter should be followed by a down-stream non-fibre releasing filter that will retain such particles.

9.84 If it is intended to use a filter for an extended period, the effectiveness of the process should be validated, taking into account such aspects as the microbial content of the solution, the capacity and efficacy of the filter and its housing, and the potential for growth of organisms on or through the filter. It is preferable not to use the filter for longer than one working day.

9.85 The filter should not adversely affect the solution by removal of ingredients from it, or by release of substances into it.

9.86 Due to the potential additional risks of the filtration method as compared with other sterilisation processes, a second filtration via a further sterilised micro-organism retaining filter, immediately prior to filling, may be advisable.

9.87 The time interval between sterilising a bulk solution by filtration and filling it into final containers should be kept to a defined minimum, appropriate to the conditions under which the filtered bulk is stored.

Sterilisation: Ethylene Oxide

9.88 The efficacy of ethylene oxide as a sterilant depends upon its concentration, the temperature and humidity (at low humidities or with free water in the chamber efficacy declines rapidly), the time of exposure and the extent of microbial contamination. Where other methods of sterilisation are practicable they should be used in preference to ethylene oxide.

9.89 Ethylene oxide can be used for sterilising the surfaces of glass, metals, rubber and plastics, but because of its high reactivity, it has a limited application. It should be used only after it has been confirmed that there are no deleterious effects on product or material and that no toxic reaction products are formed with the materials being sterilised.

[NOTE – Ethylene oxide is itself toxic, and explosive in some mixtures with air].

9.90 Direct contact between gas and microbial cells is essential. Organisms occluded in crystals or coated with other material may remain unaffected by the treatment. Steps should be taken to ensure even distribution of gas throughout the load.

9.91 The sterilisation treatment required in terms of gas concentration, temperature and time, can vary widely, and the nature and quantity of any packaging material can significantly affect the process. The efficacy of the selected process should be validated before it is adopted. Before exposure to gas, materials should be brought into equilibrium with the required humidity and temperature.

9.92 The effectiveness of an ethylene oxide cycle may be evidenced by its ability to kill resistant organisms and from a consideration of the physical records of the cycle.

9.93 Each sterilising cycle should be monitored with suitable biological indicators, distributed throughout each load. The information from these should form part of the batch record.

9.94 After exposure, materials should be held under suitably ventilated conditions to allow any ethylene oxide, and its reaction products, to diffuse away. Care should be taken to prevent recontamination of the sterilised goods, and a recorded check made that all biological indicators have been removed from the load.

9.95 Records should be made during each ethylene oxide sterilisation cycle of:

(a) the time taken to complete the cycle,
(b) the pressure,
(c) the temperature,
(d) the gas concentration,
(e) the humidity within the chamber.

The pressure and temperature should be recorded throughout the cycle on a chart, or by other suitable automatic means. These records should form part of the batch record.

Sterilisation: Radiation

9.96 Radiation sterilisation is used mainly for the sterilisation of heat-sensitive materials and products. Many medicinal products and some packaging materials are radiation-sensitive, so this method is permissible only when the absence of deleterious effects on the product has been confirmed experimentally.

9.97 The radiation employed may be gamma rays from a radio-isotope (e.g. Cobalt 60) or high energy electrons from an electron accelerator. Ultraviolet irradiation is not effective.

9.98 The normally accepted minimum sterilising dose is 25 KGy (2.5 megarads) although other levels may be adequate for particular purposes provided the process is validated. Care should be taken to ensure that *all* parts of the load receive a sterilising dose.

9.99 During the sterilisation procedure the radiation dose should be monitored. For this purpose established dosimetry procedures should be used, giving a quantitative measurement of the dose received by the product itself. Dosimeters should be inserted in the load in sufficient number, and close enough together to ensure that in continuous processing there are always at least two dosimeters in the chamber. Where plastics dosimeters are used they should be used within the time-limit of their calibration. Biological indicators should only be used as an additional control. The information obtained should form part of the batch record.

9.100 Care must be taken to distinguish between materials which have been irradiated and those which have not. Design of plant, and the use of radiation-sensitive discs, can ensure this. To this end each package should carry a radiation-sensitive disc to indicate whether it has been subjected to radiation treatment. These discs are not quantitative in their response and therefore cannot act as dosimeters. Their colour change can be affected by strong sunlight and age.

Finishing of Sterile Products

9.101 Ampoules should be sealed by a 'drawing-off' technique rather than by tip-sealing.

9.102 The integrity of the seal of containers should be checked by suitable procedures.

9.103 Containers sealed under vacuum should be tested for maintenance of that vacuum after an appropriate, pre-determined, delay.

9.104 Filled containers of parenteral products for administration to humans should be inspected individually. When this inspection is visual it should be done under suitable controlled conditions of illumination and background. Operators doing the inspection should pass regular eye-sight checks, with spectacles if worn, and be allowed adequate breaks from inspection.

9.105 Where automatic/electronic/photo-electric methods of inspection are used, the effectiveness of the equipment should be validated and its sensitivity monitored.

Biological and Chemical Indicators

9.106 Biological and Chemical Indicators used alone are not acceptable as proof that a sterilisation process has been effective. They will show when sterilisation has failed but not necessarily prove that the process has been successful.

9.107 *Biological Indicators*. Biological indicators (i.e. preparations of bacterial cultures, usually spores of selected resistant strains) are much less reliable than physical monitoring methods (except in Ethylene Oxide Sterilisation).

9.108 Strict precautions must be taken when handling biological indicators due to the hazard of introducing potential contaminants into an otherwise microbiologically clean area.

9.109 *Chemical Indicators*. Chemical Indicators are available for heat, ethylene oxide and radiation sterilisation, usually in the form of adhesive tapes or patches, colour spot cards, small tubes or sachets. They change colour as a result of chemical reaction brought about by the sterilisation process, but it is possible for the change to take place before the sterilising time has been completed, and hence, with the exception of plastic dosimeters used in radiation sterilisation, their unsuitability as full proof of sterilisation.

9.110 Certain other substances with melting points which coincide with the sterilisation temperature may be used as indicators in heat sterilisation. They indicate that the temperature has been reached, but not that it has been maintained, or for how long.

9.111 Radiation-sensitive colour discs, not to be confused with plastic dosimeters, are used to differentiate between packages which have been subjected to irradiation and those which have not. They are not indicators of successful sterilisation, and the monitoring of radiation sterilisation by calibrated plastic dosimeters is the only way of ensuring that the sterilising dose has been given.

Biological Tests

9.112 *Tests for Sterility*. When applied to the finished product a sterility test should be regarded as but one of a series of control measures by which sterility is assured. Compliance with the test does not guarantee sterility of the whole batch since sampling may fail to select non-sterile containers, and the culture methods used have limits to their sensitivity and will not necessarily permit growth of *all* micro-organisms. Nevertheless, sole reliance cannot always be placed on in-process tests and equipment controls.

9.113 The test for sterility is an exacting procedure and should be made only by skilled operators using aseptic techniques. Unless the testing is carefully controlled, it becomes a test of the operator and of laboratory procedues rather than of the product.

9.114 In sampling for sterility testing purposes, a batch should be regarded as a collection of sealed containers prepared in such a manner that the risk of contamination is the same for each of the units in it. (See 9.4 'Definitions').

9.115 Guidance on the *minimum* numbers of containers to be tested and on the standard methods available for testing various types of preparations for aerobic and anaerobic bacteria, and for fungi, is given in official compendia.

9.116 Containers taken as samples should be such that they are representative of the batch, ensuring that all parts of a heat sterilised load (including the potentially coolest part) and the beginning and end of an aseptically-filled batch are represented.

9.117 The method of choice for sterility testing is by membrane filtration.

9.118 Media to be used for sterility testing should be sterile, and subject to controls to demonstrate that they will support the growth of small numbers of relevant organisms and that they are in fact sterile.

9.119 When a batch fails the test the cause of failure should be investigated, and suitable remedial action taken.

9.120 Running records should be maintained of sterility test results. The frequency of any repeat testing can give an indication of the confidence to be placed in the testing procedure.

9.121 *Tests for Pyrogens*. Pyrogens may be introduced into a product from starting materials, from personnel or from equipment. Growth of micro-organisms will also cause pyrogens to develop in aqueous products.

9.122 In the manufacture of any sterile product, careful consideration should be given to the need for testing not only finished products, but also ingredients and bulk or intermediate products for pyrogens, and to the frequency of such testing. Pyrogens are a more serious hazard in larger volume injections.

9.123 Water, whether an ingredient or a Finished Product, is a particular risk. Water for Injections must be tested for pyrogens when labelled 'apyrogenic' or when filled into containers of over 15 ml. The presence of pyrogens in distilled water is usually an indication of contamination from cooling water in the still or of unsatisfactory storage before sterilisation.

9.124 Although limits are given in compendia for temperature increase in the rabbit test beyond which the batch should be failed or retested, any response outside the range normally encountered should be taken as a warning and its cause investigated.

9.125 The use of the limulus amoebocyte lysate test is valuable in monitoring bacterial endotoxin levels.

Batch Release

9.126 The decision to release a batch of sterile product for use should take account not only of the specific production records and results of tests performed on that batch, but also of information gathered before and during its manufacture from the monitoring of the environment, personnel, intermediate products, equipment and processes.

10. DRY PRODUCTS AND MATERIALS

General

10.1 The handling of dry materials and products creates problems of dust control and cross contamination, and special attention is needed in the design, maintenance and use of premises and equipment in order to overcome these problems. Wherever possible, enclosed dust-containing manufacturing systems should be employed. Separate 'dedicated' facilities may be necessary for manufacture involving highly potent, toxic or sensitising materials (See also 5.13 and Appendix 2).

10.2 Suitable environmental conditions should be maintained by installation of effective air-extraction systems, with discharge points sited to avoid contamination of other products and processes. Filtration or other systems should be installed to retain dust. The plant should be properly serviced and maintained. Care should be taken to contain any dust loosened when filters are removed or replaced and to avoid dust falling back on to product from extraction duct-work. The use of tablet and capsule de-dusting devices is recommended.

10.3 Special care should be taken to protect against contamination of the product by fragments of metal, glass or wood. The use of metal detectors is recommended. Glass equipment is to be avoided, and screens, sieves, punches and dies should be examined for wear or breakage before and after each use.

10.4 Care should be taken to guard against tablets or capsules which may lodge and remain undetected in equipment, counters, or bulk containers.

Mixing/granulation

10.5 Unless operated as a closed system, mixing, sifting and blending equipment should be fitted with dust extraction.

10.6 Critical operating parameters (e.g. time, power and temperature) for each mixing, blending and drying operation should be laid down in the Master Formula and Method, monitored during processing, and recorded in the batch records.

10.7 Filter bags fitted to fluid bed driers should not be used for different products, without being washed between use. With certain highly potent or sensitising products, bags specific to one product only should be used. Air entering the drier should be filtered. Steps should be taken to prevent cross-contamination by dust in the air leaving the drier. (see also Appendix 2).

10.8 Solutions should be made and used in a manner which minimises the risk of contamination or microbial growth.

Compression

10.9 Tablet compressing machines should be provided with effective dust control facilities and be sited to avoid product mix-up. Unless the same product is being made on each machine, or unless the compression machine itself provides its own enclosed air controlled environment, the machines should be sited in separate cubicles.

10.10 Suitable physical, procedural and labelling arrangements should be made to prevent mix-up of materials, granules and tablets.

10.11 Accurate calibrated check weighing equipment should be readily available and used for in-process monitoring of tablet weights. Procedures used should be capable of detecting out-of-limits tablets.

10.12 Tablets removed from a compressing cubicle or station for testing or other purposes should not be returned to the batch.

10.13 Tablets should be collected into clean, labelled, containers. A controlled system of label issue, use and destruction should be operated.

10.14 Rejected or discarded tablets should be placed in containers clearly identifying them as such and the quantity recorded in the Batch Manufacturing Record.

10.15 Setting up a compressing machine is a critical operation and the setting can change during operation. In-process controls should be employed to ensure that the products remain within specification.

10.16 Punches and dies should be examined for wear and compliance with specification, and a record of their use maintained.

Coating

10.17 Air supplied to coating pans for drying purposes should be filtered and of suitable quality.

10.18 Coating solutions should be made and used in a manner which will minimise the risk of microbial growth. Their preparation and use should be documented and recorded.

Hard Capsule Filling

10.19 Empty capsule shells should be regarded as Starting Materials and treated accordingly. They should be stored under conditions which will prevent drying and embrittlement or the effects of moisture.

10.20 Paragraphs 10.9 – 10.15 of 'Compression' (above), appropriately modified, also apply to hard capsule filling.

Tablet and Capsule Printing

10.21 Special care should be taken to avoid product mix-up during any printing of tablets and capsules. Where different products, or different batches of the same product, are printed at the same time, the operations should be adequately segregated.

10.22 Printing Ink should be regarded as a Starting Material and treated accordingly.

10.23 After printing, tablets and capsules should be approved by Quality Control before release for packaging or sale, even if the unprinted products have been previously shown to comply with their Specification.

10.24 Care should be taken to avoid mix-up during the inspection, sorting and polishing of capsules and tablets.

11. LIQUIDS, CREAMS AND OINTMENTS

[NOTE – This section refers to products which are not specified as sterile.]

11.1 Liquids, creams and ointments should be manufactured so as to protect the product from microbial and other contamination. The use of closed systems of manufacture and transfer is recommended where possible.

11.2 The chemical and microbiological quality of the water used should be monitored. Water should be of *at least* potable quality and have a low microbial count.

11.3 Where pipe-lines are used for delivery of ingredients or supply of bulk, care should be taken to ensure that such systems are both easy to clean and, in fact, clean. Pipework should be designed and installed so that it may be readily dismantled and cleaned.

11.4 Where pipe-lines are used to transfer bulk materials to remote holding vessels or filling machines it must be ensured that the material is, in fact, delivered to the intended vessel or machine.

11.5 Care should be taken, when bulk tanker deliveries are received, to ensure the quality and quantity of the delivery before use.

11.6 Measuring systems should be verified as accurate. Where dipsticks are used they should be used only with the particular vessel for which they have been calibrated. They should be made of suitable non-shedding, non-absorbent material (e.g. Not wood).

12. MEDICAL GASES

General

12.1 Gases, in either compressed or liquefied form, intended for medical use should be manufactured, filled, stored, distributed and documented in accordance with the general principles outlined in this Guide, appropriately interpreted to suit the special context of gaseous products. Although order, tidiness, cleanliness and security sufficient to avoid the risk of error, mix-up or contamination are required, certain recommendations given elsewhere in the Guide (for example on premises and equipment) may not always be applicable to a product which is never in direct contact with the factory environment. Nevertheless, particularly to encourage desirable attitudes towards medicinal products, areas where medical gases are filled should be maintained at an appropriate standard of decor, cleanliness and order.

12.2 All gas production plant should be continually monitored for the quality and impurity levels of the gas produced, and similar tests should be carried out on bulk storage vessels at specified regular intervals.

12.3 Gas production, treatment and filling plant should be designed, installed and maintained so as to avoid contamination of the gas. Filters are necessary after driers to prevent contamination with particles of desiccant.

12.4 The areas used for filling of medical gases should be segregated from areas used for filling gases for other (e.g. industrial) purposes. The 'medical' nature of such areas should be emphasised.

Staff

12.5 Staff employed on the production, filling and testing of medicinal gases should be made aware, and regularly reminded of, the special importance and the potential hazards to patients of their work. A form of protective clothing, which is distinctive, is a useful aid in making and emphasising these points.

Pipe-lines

12.6 Gas pipe-lines should be colour-coded to BS 1710 (Identification of Pipelines) and HTM 22 (Piped Medical Gases etc.) All gas outlets should be conspicuously marked to indicate the name of the gas supplied to the outlet. Cleaning and purging of pipe-lines should follow written procedures, and checks for the absence of cleaning agents or other contaminants should be carried out before the line is released for use.

Filling Areas

12.7 Filling areas should be of sufficient size, and have an orderly lay-out which will permit:

(a) Allocation of separate marked areas for different gases and different cylinder sizes.

(b) Clearly identifiable segregation of empty cylinders from full cylinders.

(c) Clear distinguishing of the stage reached by given cylinders (e.g. 'awaiting filling', 'filled', 'awaiting test and/or inspection', 're-leased').

The method used to achieve these various levels of segregation will depend on the nature, extent or complexity of the over-all operation, but marked-out floor areas, partitions, barriers, labels and signs should be used as appropriate.

Preparation of returned cylinders

12.8 New cylinders and cylinders returned for re-filling should be checked as clean and suitable before re-use. Cylinders returned from customers should be prepared for re-filling as follows:

(a) Cylinders due for statutory hydraulic test, or which require re-painting, or which are damaged in any way must receive the appropriate treatment before filling. If a cylinder is to be re-painted in a different colour, for use with a different gas, the old paint must be completely removed before re-painting.

(b) Old date/batch labels, and any markings applied by the customer, must be removed.

(c) Any water or debris in valve outlets must be removed by an air-jet or other suitable means before the cylinder valve is opened.

Filling

12.9 Before a cylinder is filled steps should be taken to avoid the risk of contamination of the new gas with any possibly contaminated gas remaining in the cylinder, by employing appropriate blow-down, purging and evacuation procedures. Checks should be made to ensure compliance with points 12.8 (a), (b) and (c) above, and in particular to ensure that the cylinder is colour-coded (ref. BS 1319 1976), labelled, stencilled or otherwise marked in accordance with the nature of the gas to be filled.

Lot Identification

12.10 In addition to identification labelling or marking, all filled cylinders should have attached a lot-identifying label. If, because of the continuous nature of gas production, it is not possible to relate this directly to a bulk-batch of gas, it should at least be indicative of date, time and place of filling, and permit access to a relevant test-record.

Release

12.11 Following filling, all cylinders should be leak-tested by an appropriate method, and held in quarantine until released by Quality Control, after checks have been made to ensure:–

(a) that all necessary tests have been carried out, and that the recorded results are within specification.

(b) that the cylinders:
- (i) have not exceeded hydraulic test date
- (ii) are in good condition and correctly painted
- (iii) are properly identity- and batch- labelled and stencilled

(c) and that:
- (i) the valve is in good condition
- (ii) any protective cap or sleeve over the out-let has been properly applied.

12.12 Whilst the general spirit of this Guide is applicable to the quality control of medical gases, it is not normally necessary or appropriate to retain finished product samples.

Storage

12.13 Gas cylinders should be stored under cover, and not subjected to extremes of temperature. Areas where they are stored should be clean, dry, well ventilated and free of combustible materials.

12.14 Storage arrangements should permit segregation of different gases and of full/empty cylinders and permit rotation of stock.

12.15 Cylinders should be stored so that they remain clean, dry and with their markings un-obscured.

12.16 Storage arrangement for gas-mixtures should be such as to avoid separation of the mixture into its component gases.

13. MANUFACTURE OF RADIOPHARMACEUTICALS

13.1 A radiopharmaceutical is a medicinal product which achieves its purpose at least in part, by virtue of its radioactivity. It may be formulated in any of the pharmaceutical presentations covered by this Guide and the general and specific guidance given should be followed as appropriate. The radioactivity may necessitate modification of this guidance in some respects.

13.2 In the manufacture of *sterile* radiopharmaceuticals the need for modification of guidance given elsewhere is likely to be most apparent. Non-radioactive components should be prepared as described in Section 9. It may be necessary to handle radioactive materials in a contained work station operated at an air-pressure *below* that of the room in which it is sited. Air admitted to the room should still have passed through terminal filters of appropriate porosity so that with the operator present and work in progress, the required class conditions (see Section 9) are maintained at the point of greatest risk, where products are exposed. All operations up to the stage of sterilisation should be carried out in a manner which minimises microbial and particulate contamination.

13.3 Because of a short useful 'life', it may be necessary to despatch products before all tests are completed. This does not reduce the need for a formal recorded decision to be taken by an authorised person as to whether or not a product should be released, based on the production and quality control data available at the time. Specifications should define at what stage of testing a decision on release may be taken.

13.4 Sterile products of short half-life radionuclides are commonly prepared by aseptic technique at or near the place of use from previously prepared components ('kits'), and the eluate of a radionuclide generator. It may be acceptable to carry out this work under environmental conditions of a lower grade than those described for aseptic work in Section 9 when the following situation pertains:

(i) the preparation is done entirely by transference of materials between closed containers, for example by use of a syringe and hypodermic needle penetrating a rubber closure, (so-called 'closed procedures').

(ii) manipulations are performed within a contained work station which, whilst giving the required degree of operator protection, also maintains the critical working zone at the standard of Grade 1A, Appendix 1.

and (iii) the product is to be administered within a few hours of preparation.

(See also 'Guidance Notes for Hospitals on the Premises and Environment for the Preparation of Radiopharmaceuticals').

Part Three

14. CONTRACT MANUFACTURE, ANALYSIS AND SERVICING

PRINCIPLES

The relative responsibilities of the Contract Giver and the Contract Acceptor (see Glossary) should be clearly understood and agreed, with the object of avoiding misunderstandings which could result in a product or work of unsatisfactory quality. In contract manufacture the Contract Giver bears the ultimate responsibility for ensuring that the product specification complies with relevant legal requirements, that the product as manufactured meets that specification, and that the specified quality is maintained during storage, transport and distribution.

Manufacture

14.1 A Contract Giver should assure himself that the Contract Acceptor has adequate premises, equipment, and staff with sufficient knowledge and experience, to carry out satisfactorily the work placed with him. In order to do this the Contract Giver should visit the Contract Acceptor's premises, both before and at times during the manufacture of his product.

14.2 A Contract Acceptor should have premises, equipment, knowledge and experience sufficient to carry out satisfactorily the work placed by a Contract Giver, and refrain from any activity which may adversely affect products manufactured for a Contract Giver.

14.3 The technical arrangements made in connection with a contract should be in writing. The limits of the responsibilities accepted by each of the parties should be clearly laid down.

14.4 Any change in technical arrangements should be agreed by both parties and should be laid down in writing.

14.5 The parties to a manufacturing contract should each appoint competent persons to:

(a) Draw up the technical arrangements for manufacture.

(b) Agree arrangements for in-process control tests and for testing Finished Products.

(c) Define the mechanism by which a batch is released for sale after review of the manufacturing, packaging and analytical records.

14.6 A Contract Acceptor should not pass to a third party any of the work entrusted to him by a Contract Giver without the latter having evaluated the arrangements and given his consent.

14.7 Arrangements made with a third party should ensure that the exchange of information is on the same basis as between the original Contract Giver and Contract Acceptor.

14.8 If a Contract Giver supplies materials, the Contract Acceptor should be given the appropriate Material Specifications. If this is not possible for reasons of commercial or research confidentiality, he should be given sufficient information to enable him to process the material correctly, and details of:

(a) Any potential hazard to premises, plant, personnel, or to other materials or products.

(b) The legal status of the materials and resultant products.

14.9 If a Contract Acceptor supplies materials, the Contract Giver should specify the quality required.

14.10 A Contract Acceptor should check that all products or materials delivered to him are suitable for the purpose intended.

14.11 A Contract Giver should ensure that all products or materials delivered to him by the Contract Acceptor comply with their Specifications. If products are delivered directly from a Contract Acceptor to the market, the Contract Giver should provide for this check to be made before they are released for sale.

14.12 If the manufacturing processes take place in two or more countries, care should be taken to ensure that whilst meeting the requirements of one country, the product still meets the requirements of the other country or countries.

14.13 Manufacturing and analytical records and reference samples should be kept by, or be readily available to, the Contract Giver. The documents kept should facilitate recall from sale of any batch of the product.

Contract Analysis

14.14 As appropriate the above provisions should apply also to contract analysis (see also under Contract Analysis in Section 8, 'Good Control Laboratory Practice').

Service Contracts

14.15 Where service or maintenance work is performed (e.g. on manufacturing or test equipment, sterilisers, controlled air supply systems) the Contract Giver should assure himself that the Contract Acceptor has sufficient equipment, staff, knowledge and experience to carry out the work.

14.16 There should be a written contract which should clearly specify the work to be carried out, and the form and detail of the report or certification required. The report or certificate should state clearly what work was done and the results achieved, and declare whether or not the equipment performs in compliance with specification.

15. VETERINARY MEDICINES

15.1 Medicinal products for veterinary use should be manufactured in accordance with the principles outlined in this Guide, but because of their nature and use, it may be appropriate to manufacture certain veterinary products under conditions differing in detail from those recommended for equivalent products intended for human use. Some veterinary products such as those used for mass external treatment of animals (e.g. sheep dips), have no direct equivalent amongst products for human use and the recommendations on manufacturing premises and equipment given elsewhere in the Guide may not be appropriate. Sufficient order, tidiness, cleanliness and security is however always required in order to minimise the risk of formulation error, mix-up and contamination.

15.2 In the manufacture of terminally sterilised veterinary products particular attention should be given to the need to minimise microbiological contamination of the product before sterilisation. Areas used for the preparation of these products should be protected from air-borne contamination from their surroundings, any artificial ventilation being through filters. The rooms should be designed and constructed in a manner which facilitates effective cleaning, and they should be maintained in a clean and tidy condition.

15.3 Areas used for filling products to be terminally sterilised should be maintained at a positive air pressure in relation to their surroundings, with a supply of filtered air. The filling operation, where products or cleaned empty containers are exposed, should be carried out in an atmosphere complying in terms of cleanliness with Grade 3 (Appendix 1) achieved either by general ventilation or by appropriate local protection (e.g. a contained work station).

15.4 Products which are not sterilised in their final containers but which are filled under aseptic conditions should be processed as described in those paragraphs relevant to aseptic processing in Section 9.

16. ELECTRONIC DATA PROCESSING

PRINCIPLES

The introduction of Electronic Data Processing into systems of manufacturing, storage and distribution does not alter the need to observe the relevant principles, given elsewhere in the Guide. Where Electronic Data Processing replaces a manual operation in a system there should be no resultant increase in the risk of a wrong or defective product reaching the user.

TERMS

Electronic Data Processing (EDP) The activity of receiving data and electronically generating from it information to be used either for reporting or for automatic control.

Computer For the purpose of this section a computer is a device designed to carry out Electronic Data Processing. The term thus encompasses the field from main-frame computers to micro-processors.

System Is used in the sense of a regulated pattern of interacting activities and techniques which are united to form an organised whole.

16.1 The responsibilities of key personnel described in the Guide are not changed by the use of computers, and it is essential that there is the closest co-operation between Production, Quality Control and Electronic Data Processing Departments. Persons in responsible positions should have appropriate training for the tasks assigned to them, including that necessary for the management of systems within their field of responsibility which utilise computers. This should include ensuring that appropriate expertise is available and used to provide advice on aspects of computer installation and operation.

16.2 A general description of the system should be produced and kept up-to-date. It should describe the principles and main features of the way in which the computer is used and how it interacts with other systems and procedures.

16.3 Before a system using a computer is brought into use it should be tested and confirmed as being capable of achieving desired results. If a manual system is being replaced it is advisable to run the two in parallel for a time, as part of this testing and validation.

16.4 Systems should be designed to take into account the need for checks, at appropriate intervals, for correct operation.

16.5 Alterations to a system or to a computer programme should only be made in accordance with a defined procedure which should include provision for checking, approving and implementing the change. Such an alteration should only be implemented with the agreement of the person responsible for the part of the system concerned, and the alteration should be recorded.

16.6 Data should only be entered or amended by persons authorised to do so. Suitable methods of deterring unauthorised entry of data include the use of keys, pass cards, personal codes and restricted access to computer terminals. There should be a defined procedure for the issue, cancellation and alteration of authorisation to amend data, including the changing of personal codes.

16.7 When critical data are being entered in a record (for example, the weight and batch number of an ingredient during dispensing) there should be an independent check on the accuracy of the record which is made.

16.8 Any alteration to an entry of critical data should be authorised and recorded with the reason for the change. Authority to alter entered data should be restricted to nominated persons.

16.9 The method of final release of a batch for sale or supply should uniquely identify the person effecting that release.

16.10 It should be possible to obtain printed copies of electronically stored data.

16.11 Data which forms part of a batch record should be securely stored against wilful or accidental damage by personnel or by physical or electronic means and in accordance with para 3.43.

16.12 Stored data should be checked for accessibility, durability and accuracy, especially after any relevant changes have been made to the computer equipment or its programmes.

16.13 There should be available adequate back-up arrangements for systems which need to be operated in the event of a break-down. The time required to bring the back-up arrangements into use should be related to the possible urgency of the need to use them. (For example, information required to effect a recall must be available at short notice.)

16.14 The procedures to be followed if the system fails or breaks down should be defined and tested. Any failures and remedial action taken should be recorded.

16.15 A procedure should be established to record and analyse errors and to enable improvements to be made.

16.16 When outside agencies are used to provide a computer service there should be a formal agreement including a clear statement of the responsibilities of that outside agency. (see Section 14).

17. HOMOEOPATHIC MEDICINES

17.1 Homoeopathic products and other non-allopathic, minute-dose preparations should be manufactured and controlled in accordance with the principles outlined in this Guide.

17.2 In cases of difficulty in applying analytical tests to the final product, controls on raw materials and intermediates, in-process checks and manufacturing documentation are of particular importance.

18. GOOD PHARMACEUTICAL WHOLESALING PRACTICE

General

18.1 The recommendations of the other relevant sections of this Guide in relation to buildings, pest control, stock records and stock rotation should be followed. The warehouse, storage areas and surroundings should be maintained in a clean and tidy condition, free from accumulated waste. Spilled substances should be promptly cleaned up and rendered safe.

18.2 Key personnel involved in the warehousing of medicinal products should have the ability and experience appropriate to the responsibility of ensuring that the products or materials are properly handled.

18.3 Stocks should be received in a separate reception area, and examined for correctness against order, and for absence of damaged containers.

18.4 Medicinal Products should be stored apart from other goods where there is any risk of mix-up, or of harmful cross contamination by, or of, the other goods.

18.5 All products should be protected from excessive local heating, and from undue exposure to direct sunlight, and (unless they are known to be unaffected) from freezing.

18.6 Special storage facilities should be provided as necessary to protect products from deterioration and to comply with manufacturers' directions and with legal requirements.

18.7 Refrigerated storage areas should be equipped with temperature recorders or other devices that will indicate when the specified temperature range has not been maintained. Control should be adequate to maintain all parts of the storage area within the specified temperature range.

18.8 There should be a system to ensure stock rotation, with regular and frequent checks that the system is operating correctly. Products beyond their expiry date or shelf-life should be removed from usable stock and neither sold nor supplied.

18.9 Stock which is damaged or withheld from supply, and which is not immediately destroyed, should be kept apart from saleable stock, so that it cannot be sold in error, and so that leakage from any broken package cannot contaminate other goods.

18.10 Stocks of supposedly sterile products with broken seals, damaged packaging, or suspected of possible contamination must not be sold or supplied.

18.11 Products should be transported in such a way that:

(a) The identification of the product is not lost.

(b) The product does not contaminate, and is not contaminated by, other products or materials.

(c) Adequate precautions are taken against spillage or breakage.

(d) The product and its pack are not subjected to unacceptable degrees of heat, cold, light, moisture or other adverse influence, nor to attack by micro-organisms or pests.

18.12 Medicinal Products requiring controlled temperature storage should also be transported by appropriately specialised means.

18.13 Goods which have been rejected, recalled or returned should be placed in adequately segregated storage to avoid confusion with other materials and products and prevent redistribution, until a decision has been reached as to their disposition.

18.14 The means of recalling products should be documented (see Section 7) and records of any recalled products received into the warehouse should be kept.

Returned Goods

18.15 Goods which have left the care of the wholesale dealer should only be returned to saleable stock if:

(a) The goods are in their original unopened containers and in good condition,

(b) It is known that the goods have not been subject to adverse conditions,

(c) They have been examined and assessed by a person authorised to do so. This assessment should take into account the nature of the product, any special storage conditions it requires, and the time elapsed since it was issued. As necessary, advice should be sought from the person responsible for the Quality Control of the manufactured product.

Records

18.16 Clear, readily available records of each sale should be made, showing date of supply, customer, product name and quantity. They should be retained until at least the end of the shelf life, or the anticipated use-life, of the product concerned. A record should also be kept of the dates between which particular batches of large volume infusion fluids, vaccines and sera have been supplied.

Appendix 1
BASIC ENVIRONMENTAL STANDARDS FOR THE MANUFACTURE OF STERILE PRODUCTS

Grade	Final Filter Efficiency (as determined by BS 3928)[1]	Recommended Minimum Air Changes per hour	Max. permitted number of particles per cubic metre equal to or above:[2]		Max. permitted No. of viable organisms per cubic metre[2,3]	Nearest Equivalent Standard Classification		
			0.5 micron	5 micron		BS 5295[4]	US Fed. Std. 209B[5]	VDI 2083, P.1[6]
1/A (Unidirectional air flow work station)	99.997%	flow of 0.3m/s (vertical) or 0.45m/s (horizontal)	3000	0	less than 1	1	100	—
1/B	99.995%	20	3000	0	5	1	100	3
2	99.95%	20	300 000	2000	100	2	10 000	5
3	95.0%	20	3500 000	20 000	500	3	100 000	6

Air pressure should always be highest in the area of greatest risk to product. The air pressure differentials between rooms of successively higher to lower risk should be at least 1.5 mm (0.06 inch) water gauge.

[1] BS 3928: Method for Sodium Flame Test for Air Filters, British Standards Institution, London, 1969.

[2] This condition should be achieved throughout the room when unmanned, and recovered within a short 'clean up' period after personnel have left. The condition should be maintained in the zone immediately surrounding the product whenever the product is exposed. (Note: It is accepted that it may not always be possible to demonstrate conformity with *particulate* standards at the point of fill, with filling in progress, due to generation of particles or droplets from the product itself).

[3] Mean values obtained by air sampling methods.

[4] BS 5295: Environmental Cleanliness in Enclosed Spaces, British Standards Institution, London, 1976.

[5] US Federal Standard 209B, 1973.

[6] Verein Deutscher Ingenieure 2083, P.1.

Appendix 2
CONTROL OF CROSS-CONTAMINATION

1. The risk of cross-contamination arises from the uncontrolled release of dust, gases, vapours, sprays or organisms from materials and products in process, from residues in equipment, and from operators' clothing. Its significance varies with the type of contaminant. The most hazardous are potent low-dose materials, sensitising agents, cytotoxic materials and some living organisms.

2. Facilities, procedures (and, as necessary air-flow rates and directions) should be such as to minimise the risk of cross contamination, although the precautions which need to be taken vary according to the type of potential contamination.

3. As necessary, cross contamination should be controlled by some or all of the following measures:

(a) processing and filling in segregated areas;

(b) avoiding manufacture of different products at the same time unless they are effectively segregated;

(c) containment of material-transfer by means of air-locks, air extraction, clothing change and careful washing and decontamination of equipment;

(d) Protecting against the risks of contamination caused by recirculation of untreated air, or by inadvertent re-entry of extracted air.

(e) The use of 'closed-systems' of manufacture.

[Note – Where the starting material is an animal tissue it is important to ensure that the final stages of processing, and the end-product itself, are segregated from the starting materials].

4. Ineffective cleaning of equipment is a common source of cross-contamination, and cleaning procedures of known effectiveness should be used. Particular attention should be given to the cleaning of pipelines, valves, joints, bearings, blanked-off ends, and drying, milling, sieving and blending equipment.

5. Protective clothing worn in an area of special risk should not be worn outside it, and should be laundered in such a place and manner that contamination is contained.

6. Ovens and other equipment should only contain one product at a time.

7. Procedures should especially be established for monitoring likely contamination by potent low-dose and sensitising agents. (See also Section 10, 'Dry Products and Materials').

Appendix 3
CERTIFICATES OF ANALYSIS

1. In certain circumstances, compliance with the starting material specification may be demonstrated *in part* by possession of an acceptable Certificate of Analysis. For such a certificate to be considered acceptable, the following conditions should apply:

(a) The person responsible for Quality Control in the purchasing company must assure himself that the organisation issuing the certificate is competent to do so, whether that organisation is part of the supplying company or is independent of it (e.g. is a contract analytical service).

(b) The certificate must:

- (i) Identify the organisation issuing it, be signed by a person competent to do so, and indicate his qualifications.
- (ii) Name the material to which it refers and identify it by a batch number.
- (iii) State that the material has been tested, by whom, and when this was done.
- (iv) State the specification (e.g. 'BP') and methods against which, and by which, the tests were performed.
- (v) Give the test results obtained, or declare that the results obtained showed compliance with the stated specification.

2. Certificates which merely carry such statements as 'a typical analysis is . . .', or state that the material is of a particular quality with no supporting evidence, are not acceptable.

3. Possession of a Certificate of Analysis does not eliminate the need to confirm the identity of the material supplied. (See 5.18 and Appendix 4).

4. Possession of a Certificate of Analysis does not absolve the purchaser from ultimate responsibility for the correctness of the material to which it refers.

[Note – The above paragraphs, whilst more particularly concerned with certification of starting materials, also apply as appropriate to other materials and products].

Appendix 4
ASSURANCE OF THE IDENTITY OF STARTING MATERIALS

1. The manufacturer of medicinal products must be aware of the possibility that containers of starting materials may be incorrectly labelled, and take steps to ensure that only the correct materials are used. Sampling and identity-testing the contents of each container can provide the necessary assurance, but large deliveries in many containers can present practical and economic problems. In such circumstances it may be possible to relax the policy of identity-testing the contents of every container, if account is taken of the following:

(a) The use to which the material is to be put. Every container of material intended for use as an ingredient of injectable products should normally be sampled and identified. In the light of further considerations (which follow) it may not be necessary to sample and identify each container of material for use in other product categories.

(b) The range of materials produced and handled by the original producer and any subsequent agents. The hazards of mis-labelling are markedly reduced if the supplier deals only in one product or type of product. It is likely to be small if the supplier deals only in food products, greater if the supplier deals in a wide range of pharmaceutical materials, and probably greater still if the supplier deals in materials for both the Pharmaceutical and other industries. The broker who breaks and re-packages bulk material may well represent a high level of risk.

(c) The status of the supplying company, its history of reliability and the purchasing company's own assessment of its Quality Assurance systems and procedures.

(d) Whether or not the pharmaceutical manufacturer's own manufacturing and Quality Control procedures, including assays of the end-product, would reveal the use of a wrong material (eg where a material is assayed in the finished product and the assay is specific).

(e) Whether or not a process would self-evidently fail if the wrong material was used.

[NOTE – This Appendix, which is based on the statement which appeared in Medicines Act Information Letter ['MAIL'] No. 22 of December 1978, paragraphs 19–22, refers only to sampling for identification purposes and not to sampling for quality and compliance with specification].

Appendix 5
AVOIDANCE OF MISLABELLING AND SIMILAR ERRORS

1. Mislabelling (or the mis-use, mis-application or mix-up of other printed materials) is the most frequent cause of product hazard and product recall. Constant care and attention should be given to preventing such errors at all stages.

2. Measures which will help to avoid labelling errors include:

(a) Training staff in the special care needed in the handling and use of printed packaging materials. Such training should be extended not only to the production staff directly concerned with packaging, but also to all others involved in the design, preparation, acquisition, storage, issue and transportation of printed materials.

(b) Secure storage and transportation, both within and without the factory.

(c) An understanding (from first-hand knowledge) by the pharmaceutical manufacturer of his printer's facilities and procedures, and of the precautions taken in the print-shop to avoid mix-up at source. Agreements should be reached as to the means of preventing such mix-ups (eg limitations on the numbers and types of labels which may be gang-printed on the one sheet, segregation of different printing operations, manner of packing bulk labels, precautions during label-cutting and storage, identification of printing plates, blocks and the like).

(d) Taking care to ensure that there is no 'casual' issue of labels etc and that they are only issued by and to authorised persons.

(e) Issue of known numbers of labels and reconciliation of usage.

(f) Thorough packaging line clearance and check procedures.

(g) On-line batch coding (as distinct from batch-coding in a print shop).

(h) Use of label code readers and label and pack counters.

(i) Use of roll-feed labels and electronic scanning of them before use, or on line, paying particular attention to labels on either side of any splice.

(j) Making visual checks during a packaging run (whether or not electronic devices are used), with independent quality control checks during or at the end of the run. The results of such checks should form part of the Batch Packaging Record.

(k) Designing and printing labels and other printed materials to give marked differentiation between products (eg different sizes, different shapes, different colours).

GLOSSARY OF SOME TERMS USED IN THIS GUIDE

Analytical Method A detailed description of the procedures to be followed in performing tests for conformity with a Specification.

Batch A defined quantity of material, or bulk, intermediate or finished product that is intended or purported to be uniform in character and quality, and which has been produced during a defined cycle of manufacture. To complete certain stages of manufacture it may be necessary to divide a batch into a number of sub-batches, which are later brought together to form a final uniform batch.

A batch is sometimes described as a lot.

Batch Number (or Lot Number) A distinctive combination of numbers and/or letters which specifically identifies a batch or lot and permits its history to be traced.

Batch Manufacturing Record A document stating the materials used and the operations carried out during the processing of a given batch, including details of in-process controls, but normally excluding packaging information. It should be based on the Master Formula and Method and be compiled as the manufacturing operation proceeds.

Batch Packaging Record A document stating the bulk product and packaging materials used, and the processes carried out during the packaging of a given batch, with details of in-process controls. It should be based on the Master Packaging Instruction and be compiled during the packaging operation.

Bulk Product Any product which has completed all processing stages up to, but not including, packaging.

Contract Manufacture, Analysis or Servicing — Manufacture (or partial manufacture), Analysis or Service Work ordered by one person or organisation (the Contract Giver) and carried out by an independent person or organisation (the Contract Acceptor).

Dedicated Facility — A room or suite or rooms with attendant equipment and services (including air-supply as necessary) used only for the manufacture of one product, or a closely related group of products. (Equipment may be similarly 'dedicated').

Documentation — All the written production procedures, instructions and records, quality control procedures, and recorded test results involved in the manufacture of a medicinal product.

Finished Product — A medicinal product which has undergone all stages of manufacture, including packaging.

Good Manufacturing Practice — See Section 1.

In-Process Control — Tests, checks and measurements made during the course of manufacture (including packaging) to ensure that the resultant product will comply with its specification. Tests applied to the environment or to equipment, as well as to products in process, may be regarded as a part of in-process control.

Intermediate Product — A partly processed material which must undergo further processing before it becomes a Bulk or Finished Product.

Manufacture — The complete cycle of production of a medicinal product from the acquisition of all materials through all processing and subsequent packaging to the despatch for sale or supply of the finished product. (Unless the context otherwise requires, manufacture includes packaging).

Master Formula and Method — A document stating the starting materials, with their quantities, to be used in the manufacture of a medicinal product, together with a description of the manufacturing operations including details of specific in-process controls, but normally excluding packaging information.

Master Packaging Instruction — A document listing the components to be used for a stated container or package together with a description of the method of packaging and with details of specific in-process controls. The Instructions should include the method of assembling the component parts, if the package is complex.

Medicinal Product As defined in the Medicines Act 1968, or regulations made under it.

Monitor To monitor a process or a situation is to carry out repeated measurements or observations of one or more characteristics of the process or situation to determine whether or not it is continuing as intended. Monitoring may be continuous or intermittent and not necessarily performed on every batch.

Packaging Material Any material used in the packaging of a product. The term is not normally extended to cover the outer packaging or delivery cases used for the transportation or shipment of orders. Note – There are various categories of packaging materials, eg

(a) Packaging materials which come in contact with the product (often called 'Primary Packaging Materials').

(b) Printed packaging materials.

(c) Other packaging materials.

Although these categories are not necessarily mutually exclusive, the nature and extent of the control which needs to be applied to them may vary.

Patient Includes both human and other animals.

Processing Stages The separate operations (or groups of related operations) involved in the manufacture of a medicinal product.

Quality The essential nature of a thing and the totality of its attributes and properties which bear upon its fitness for its intended purpose.

Quality Assurance See Section 1.

Quality Control See Section 1.

Quarantine The status of materials, intermediates or products set apart whilst awaiting a decision on their suitability for processing, or for sale or distribution.

Specification A document giving a description of a starting material, packaging material, intermediate, bulk or finished product in terms of its chemical, physical and (possibly) biological characteristics. A specification normally includes descriptive clauses and numerical clauses, the latter stating standards and permitted tolerances.

Standard Operating Procedure (S.O.P.) A written authorised procedure which gives instructions for performing operations not necessarily specific to a given product or material, but of a more general nature (eg equipment operation, maintenance and cleaning; cleaning of premises and environmental control; sampling and inspection etc). Certain Standard Operating Procedures may be used to supplement the product-specific Master and Batch production documentation.

Starting Material Any substance used in the manufacture of a medicinal product, but excluding packaging materials. A starting material is sometimes known as a *raw material* or an *ingredient*, although not all starting materials necessarily remain as ingredients of the final product.

Status The classification of any goods, materials, containers or machines in relation to their acceptance (or otherwise) for use, further processing or distribution (eg 'Quarantine', 'On Test', 'Released', 'Restricted Use', 'Hold', 'Rejected', 'Clean', 'To be Cleaned').

Status Label A label applied to a material, product, container or machine indicative of its status.

Sterility The complete absence of living organisms.

[NOTE – The state of sterility is an absolute. There are no degrees of sterility].

Sterile That which is in a state of sterility.

Sterilise To render sterile.

Validation The action of proving that any material, process, procedure, activity, system, equipment or mechanism used in manufacture or control can, will and does achieve the desired and intended result(s).

SELECT BIBLIOGRAPHY
A. UK ACTS REGULATIONS AND ORDERS

Medicines Act 1968 (HMSO 1968)

Medicines Act 1971 (HMSO 1971)

Regulations and Orders (Pub. HMSO) made under Medicines Act 1968:

SI 1971 No.972	The Medicines (Standard Provisions for Licences and Certificates) Regulations 1971
SI 1971 No.973	The Medicines (Applications for Product Licences, Clinical Trial Certificates and Animal Test Certificates) Regulations 1971
SI 1971 No.974	The Medicines (Applications for Manufacturer's and Wholesale Dealer's Licences) Regulations 1971
SI 1971 No.1200	The Medicines (Control of Substances for Manufacture) Order 1971
SI 1971 No.1450	The Medicines (Exemption from Licences) (Special and Transitional Cases) Order 1971
SI 1972 No.1200	The Medicines (Exemption from Licences) (Special Cases and Miscellaneous Provisions) Order 1972
SI 1972 No.1201	The Medicines (Applications for Product Licences and Clinical Trial and Animal Test Certificates) Amendment Regulations 1972

SI 1972 No.1226	The Medicines (Standard Provisions for Licences and Certificates) Amendment Regulations 1972
SI 1973 No.367	The Medicines (Extension to Antimicrobial Substances) Order 1973
SI 1974 No.1150	The Medicines (Exemption from Licences) (Ingredients) Order 1974
SI 1974 No.1523	The Medicines (Standard Provisions for Licences and Certificates) Amendment Regulations 1974
SI 1975 No.681	The Medicines (Applications for Product Licences and Clinical Trial and Animal Test Certificates) Amendment Regulations 1975
SI 1976 No.1726	The Medicines (Labelling) Regulations 1976
SI 1977 No.675	The Medicines (Standard Provisions for Licences and Certificates) Amendment Regulations 1977
SI 1977 No. 996	The Medicines (Labelling) Amendment Regulations 1977
SI 1977 No.1039	The Medicines (Standard Provisions for Licences and Certificates) Amendment (No.2) Regulations 1977
SI 1977 No.1050	The Medicines (Medicines Act 1968 Amendment) Regulations 1977
SI 1977 No.1051	The Medicines (Applications for Product Licences and Clinical Trial and Animal Test Certificates) Amendment Regulations 1977
SI 1977 No.1052	The Medicines (Applications for Manufacturer's and Wholesale Dealer's Licences) Amendment Regulations 1977
SI 1977 No.1053	The Medicines (Standard Provisions for Licences and Certificates) Amendment (No.3) Regulations 1977

SI 1977 No.1054	The Medicines (Exemption from Licences) (Wholesale Dealing) Order 1977
SI 1977 No.1399	The Medicines (Certificate of Analysis) Regulations 1977
SI 1977 No.1488	The Medicines (Breathing Gases) Order 1977
SI 1977 No.2168	The Medicines (Labelling) Amendment (No.2) Regulations 1977
SI 1978 No.1138	The Medicines (Intra-Uterine Contraceptive Devices) (Appointed Day) Order 1978
SI 1978 No.1139	The Medicines (Intra-Uterine Contraceptive Devices) (Amendment to Exemption from Licences) Order 1978
SI 1978 No.1140	The Medicines (Licensing of Intra-Uterine Contraceptive Devices) (Miscellaneous Amendments) Regulations 1978
SI 1979 No.1539	The Medicines (Contact Lens Fluids and Other Substances) (Appointed Day) Order 1979
SI 1979 No.1585	The Medicines (Contact Lens Fluids and Other Substances) (Exemption from Licences) Order 1979
SI 1979 No.1745	The Medicines (Contact Lens Fluids and Other Substances) (Exemption from Licences) Amendment Order 1979
SI 1979 No.1759	The Medicines (Contact Lens Fluids and Other Substances) (Labelling) Regulations 1979
SI 1979 No.1760	The Medicines (Contact Lens Fluids and Other Substances) (Advertising and Miscellaneous Amendments) Regulations 1979
SI 1981 No.1689	The Medicines (Contact Lens Fluids and Other Substances) (Labelling) Amendment Regulations 1981

SI 1981 No.1791 The Medicines (Labelling) Amendment Regulations 1981

B. EUROPEAN COMMUNITY DIRECTIVES

65/65/EEC
Council Directive of 26 January 1965 on the approximation of provisions laid down by law, regulation or administrative action relating to proprietary medicinal products (Official Journal of the European Communities 9.2.65, pp. 369–373).

75/319/EEC*
Second Council Directive of 20 May 1975 on the approximation of provisions laid down by law, regulation or administrative action relating to proprietary medicinal products (Official Journal of the European Communities 9.6.75, L 147, pp. 13–22).

*This Directive sets out requirements for the Qualified Person

C. MEDICINES ACT LEAFLETS ('MAL')

The following are some of the leaflets, giving information on various aspects of medicines legislation, which are available from Medicines Division, DHSS.

MAL 1 Guide to the Licensing System (Revised December 1976)

MAL 2 Notes on Applications for Product Licences (Medicines for Human Use) (Revised February 1983)

MAL 5 Notes on applications for Manufacturer's Ordinary Licences (1971)

MAL 6 Notes on applications for Wholesale Dealer's Licences. (Revised June 1979)

MAL 18 Licensing Requirements involved in the Packaging and Labelling of Medicinal Products. (Revised September 1980)

MAL 21 Notes on licensing of Homoeopathic Products (Revised November 1982)

MAL 22 Application of the Act to Ingredients. (Revised August 1974)

MAL 41 Additional Notes for Guidance – Biological Medicinal Products (Revised May 1982)

MAL 42 Notes on the Medicines (Labelling) Regulations 1976 (1976)

MAL 44 Implementation of EEC Directives about the Marketing and Manufacture of Medicinal Products (1977)

MAL 45 Notes on European Community Requirements about the 'Qualified Person' (Revised February 1982)

MAL 46 Notes on European Community Requirements for the Importation of Proprietary Medicinal Products (For Human Use) (Revised January 1982)

MAL 49 Notes on the Medicines (Labelling) Amendment Regulations 1977 (1977)

MAL 59 Hearings and Representations under Part II of the Medicines Act 1968 (1979)

MAL 99 The Control of Medicines in the United Kingdom of Great Britain and Northern Ireland (Revised June 1981)

Requests for copies should be addressed to the Department of Health and Social Security, Medicines Division, Market Towers, 1 Nine Elms Lane, London, SW8 5NQ.

[NOTE – A Medicines Act Information Letter – 'MAIL' – is issued as an occasional publication of Medicine Division DHSS, to UK Licence Holders. See in particular MAIL 22 of December 1978 paras. 19–22, on Sampling and Identification of Raw Materials].

D. BRITISH STANDARDS (Pub. British Standards Institution, 2 Park Street, London W1A 2BS)

BS 1319: 1976 Specification for Medical Gas Cylinders, Valves and Yoke Connections

1319C: 1976 Chart of Colours for the Identification of the Contents of Medical Gas Cylinders

BS 1710: 1975 Identification of Pipelines

BS 3421: 1961 Performance of Electrically Heated Sterilising Ovens

BS 3928: 1969 Method for Sodium Flame Test for Air Filters

BS 3970: —— Steam Sterilisers:

BS 3970: Part 1: 1966 Sterilisers for Porous Loads

BS 3970: Part 2: 1966 Sterilisers for Bottled Fluids

BS 3970: Part 5: 1968 Electrically Heated Steam Generators for use with Hospital Sterilisers

BS 4778: 1979 Glossary of Terms used in Quality Assurance (including Reliability and Maintainability terms)

BS 4891: 1972 A Guide to Quality Assurance

BS 5295*: ——Environmental Cleanliness in Enclosed Spaces:

BS 5295: Part 1: 1976 Specification for Controlled Environment Clean Rooms, Work Stations and Clean Air Devices

BS 5295: Part 2: 1976 Guide to the Construction and Installation of Clean Rooms, Work Stations and Clean Air Devices

BS 5295: Part 3: 1976 Guide to Operational Procedures and Disciplines applicable to Clean Air Devices

BS 5726: 1979 Specification for Microbiological Safety Cabinets

BS 5750: —— Quality Systems:

BS 5750: Part 1: 1979 Specification for Design, Manufacture and Installation

BS 5750: Part 2: 1979	Specification for Manufacture and Installation
BS 5750: Part 3: 1979	Specification for Final Inspection and Test
BS 5750: Part 4: 1981	Guide to use of BS 5750, Part 1
BS 5750: Part 5: 1981	Guide to use of BS 5750, Part 2
BS 5750: Part 6: 1981	Guide to use of BS 5750, Part 3

*See also US Federal Standard 209B (Clean Room and Work Station Requirements, Controlled Environment) and Verein Deutscher Ingenieure 2083, P.I.

E. OTHER PUBLICATIONS

Department of Health and Social Security. Sterilisers. (Health Technical Memorandum 10) London, HMSO, 1980

Department of Health and Social Security. Piped medical gases, medical compressed air and medical vacuum installations. (Health Technical Memorandum 22) London, HMSO, 1977

Department of Health and Social Security. Guidance Notes for Hospitals on Premises and Environment for the Preparation of Radiopharmaceuticals. London, DHSS, 1982.

Pharmaceutical Society. Guidelines for the handling of cytotoxic drugs. *Pharmaceutical Journal*, 1983, vol. 230, pp. 230–231.

Parenteral Drug Association, Inc.: Validation of steam sterilisation cycles. (Technical Monograph No.1) Philadelphia, P.D.A., 1978

Parenteral Drug Association, Inc.: Validation of aseptic filling for solution drug products. (Technical Monograph No.2) Philadelphia, P.D.A., 1980

Parenteral Drug Association, Inc.: Validation of dry heat processes used for sterilisation and depyrogenation. (Technical Report No.3) Philadelphia, P.D.A., 1981

INDEX

Printed in the United Kingdom for Her Majesty's Stationery Office
Dd289653 11/87 C30 8206